KT-524-008

Contents

PART 3 Get Fatburning Now

PART 4 Fatburning Menus and Recipes

Acknowledgements

This book would not have been possible without the help and support of many people. A very special thanks goes to Natalie Savona, whose help, editing, research and sculpting of recipes was invaluable; to Jan for taking care of everything else; and to Rachel Winning, my editor at Piatkus, and all her very professional and supportive team.

ABBREVIATIONS AND MEASURES

1 gram (g) = 1000 milligrams (mg) = 1,000,000 micrograms (mcg or μg)
   Most vitamins are measured in milligrams or micrograms.
   Vitamins A, D and E are also measured in International Units (iu), a measurement designed to standardise the various forms of vitamins that have different potencies.

1mcg of retinol (1mcg RE) = 3.3iu of vitamin A
1mcg RE of betacarotene = 6mcg of betacarotene
100iu of vitamin D = 2.5mcg
100iu of vitamin E = 67mg

1 pound (lb) = 16 ounces (oz), 2.2lb = 1 kilogram (kg)
1 pint = 0.6 litres, 1.76 pints = 1 litre
In this book, calories means kilocalories (kcals)

2 teaspoons (tsp) = 1 dessertspoon (dsp)
1.5 dessertspoons = 1 tablespoon (tbsp)

PART 1

Dieting Facts and Fantasies

1

What is the Fatburner Diet?

ARE YOU CONFUSED about how to lose weight? Are you having difficulty losing or maintaining weight?

In the last five years there have been some major break-throughs in the science of weight control. We now know much more about precisely what kinds of foods help you to burn fat and stay lean, thus making it easier to lose weight and gain health than ever before. We also understand more why certain types of diets fail for certain types of people. This book aims to set the record straight as far as weight control is concerned, and give you a highly practical way to lose weight by burning off excess fat.

Your Weight is a Burning Issue

If you are overweight, the chances are that your body is pro-grammed to turn food into fat, instead of energy. In the long run, simply counting calories and avoiding fat won't help. In fact, it could harm you. Your weight is a *burning* issue. Many factors in today's diet and lifestyle stop you burning fat. The good news is that we now know how you can reprogramme your body to burn fat. It only takes about 30 days. By then you are a Fatburner, and the pounds will fall off without you having to starve yourself.

The Fatburner Diet May Seriously Improve Your Health

This isn't just about weight loss. The principles of the Fatburner Diet have been proven to:

- Increase your energy.
- Stabilise and improve your mood.
- Increase your stress resistance.
- Boost your mental alertness and concentration.
- Reduce your risk of heart disease.
- Reduce your risk of diabetes.
- Burn fat.

Don't just take my word for it. Hear what was said when we invited four magazines – *The Sunday Times Magazine, Time Out, She* and *Woman's Realm* – to find volunteers and put the diet to the test.

Woman's Realm tried it out on three people: Sabine, Ian and Tina. Here's what they said: 'Sabine complained of erratic weight and constant lack of energy. She's tried loads of diets which only ever gave temporary and limited success. It was her ambition to get down to 8 stone (112lb) and stay there, plus regain some of her get-up-and-go in the process!

'Sabine reached her target weight in just a few months. Her food weaknesses – mid-morning nibbles on crisps and chocolate – have completely gone. "Once I got used to eating lots of fruit, my craving for sugar and chocolate disappeared." Sabine now says her whole attitude to food has changed. "I'm no longer obsessed with eating and automatically reach for healthy things when I shop and cook." Sabine says it's wonderful to feel so relaxed around food. She lost 10lb in three months. Her only problem was coping with the extra energy.

'Ian's weight had hovered stubbornly around the 15 stone (210lb) mark. He was also drinking and smoking heavily and wanted to reduce both significantly.

'Now only a few pounds off his target weight, Ian has managed to give up smoking and drastically reduce his alcohol consumption, a daunting task on top of his highly pressurised job as a theatre producer/actor. Ian started gradually, cutting out tea and coffee, then reducing his red meat/fried food intake. Soon he was following the diet rigorously. Once he'd lost a stone (14lb) in weight, Ian started to reduce his alcohol consumption – from two bottles of wine to two glasses per day – and eventually felt ready to stop the cigarettes, which he did overnight. Ian's comments: "I was very apprehensive at the beginning – I had a lot of vices to conquer. But once I got over my craving for caffeine it was easier to crack the weight problem." Ian lost 19lb.

'Gina's problem was willpower. Having a huge appetite and a sweet tooth for chocolate and puddings, she admitted to eating throughout the day whether she was hungry or not!

'First of all she reduced her tea and coffee intake and substituted fruit or healthy snacks for chocolate. Gradually, as she ate less food high in saturated fat (like red meat), and more fruits and vegetables, her craving for sugar and sweet things lessened. Gina lost 10lb and continues to lose 1–2lb a week.'

She magazine selected 10 volunteers. This is what they reported: 'Increased alertness was a significant benefit. By the third day, everybody felt well – alert on rising, and three of us (including me) were bounding about full of the joys of spring. Two out of 10 felt hungry, but the rest said that, as far as hunger was concerned, it was a comparatively easy diet to stick to. Mrs Kilby noted by day 4 that her concentration had improved, and this was backed up by comments from other testers. Nobody had that weak and wobbly feeling associated with dieting. By the end of the week, everyone had stayed the course. Weight loss over the week varied from 3lb to 7lb, 4–5lb being the average.'

The Sunday Times selected one volunteer. This is what they said: 'After the first few days I began to feel wonderful – alert and fit and thoroughly detoxified with no more puffy eyes staring back from the bathroom mirror. There's no shortage of recipe ideas. I lost 10lb in a month and regained 2lb on holiday, but will whittle that off by eating sensibly.'

This was *Time Out*'s comment: 'Weight loss: 4lb to 7lb in four weeks. Verdict: Makes you look and feel good. Side effects: None.'

Britain's first Fatburner said this: 'I lost 3 stone and never felt hungry. I know I'll never go back to eating like I used to.'

In truth, you can expect even better results than these. That's because the Fatburner Diet programme in this book is the result of making some major improvements to the original diet that these volunteers went on, based on recent breakthroughs in obesity research and fine-tuning the diet, based on feedback from volunteers. Are you ready for it?

What is the Fatburner Diet?

Both theory and practice of the Fatburner Diet are simple. The body burns glucose (sugar) and turns it into energy, so much of what you eat gets broken down, ultimately into glucose to make energy. When your body has more glucose than you need, the excess is put into storage as fat.

If the glucose level in your blood stays incredibly even, you will have a consistent energy level and no problem maintaining the right weight. If, on the other hand, your blood glucose level is uneven – sometimes high, sometimes low – when it is too high you turn the glucose into fat, and when it's too low you feel lethargic. One quarter of all people, and at least three-quarters of those with weight problems, have an uneven blood sugar level (technically called dysglycemia). The net consequence is that you end up fat and lethargic.

Carried to the extreme, loss of blood glucose stability leads to diabetes. Obese people are *77 times* more likely to develop diabetes than non-obese people. Weight gain and blood sugar control are strongly connected.

Cutting calories or low-fat diets may help but they are not the answer. The answer lies in reprogramming your body to burn fat by regaining blood glucose control. When this is achieved you can lose weight effortlessly without having to starve. And you also gain health and vitality at the same time.

HOW TO USE THIS BOOK

If you want to get started today go straight to Part 3: Get Fatburning Now. This explains exactly what you have to do, and is supported with suggested menus and recipes in Part 4.

Meanwhile, to truly take charge of your health, it's better to understand 'why' as well as 'how'. Part 2 explains each key factor of the 30 Day Fatburner Diet, backed up with scientific explanations.

But first, let's examine the shortfalls of other diet regimes, explode dieting myths and give you the facts about weight gain and weight loss.

2

Exploding the Myths

BEFORE WE LEARN about the key principles of the Fat-burner Diet, it helps to 'unlearn' some of the popular myths about losing weight.

Myth 1: The Only Way to Lose Weight is to Eat Less or Exercise More

Conventional opinion says that if you subtract the calories you burn off as exercise from the calories you take in as food the remainder ends up as a wad of fat around your middle. So, the only way to lose weight is to eat fewer calories or to do more exercise. While this is part of the truth, it is certainly not the whole truth.

Over the last 20 years the average calorie intake has dropped by 20 per cent – we are eating less food. Our fat intake has also dropped by 25 per cent. So we are eating fewer calories, and fewer calories as fat.[1] Yet excess weight and obesity are rocketing – incidence has almost tripled in 15 years. Currently one in three people is overweight and one in five is obese.[2] Although we are exercising less, this alone does not explain the explosion in weight gain.

Myth 2: You Can't Change Your Metabolism

Your metabolism is the process by which your body turns your food into energy or into storage as fat. We are each programmed to respond differently to the food we eat. This programming is partly inherited, but mainly the consequence of what you eat. Both the working of your metabolism and your metabolic rate – the speed at which you burn calories – can change. Crash diets can lower your metabolic rate to half-speed, while aerobic exercise can increase your metabolic rate tenfold and leave it raised for up to 15 hours. Some people's metabolism is programmed to rapidly turn food into fat. By changing the kinds and combinations of food you eat you can reprogramme yourself to burn fat more rapidly.

Myth 3: Eating Fat, Not Sugar, Makes You Fat

The fat you eat is the same fat you're sitting on. All fat, sugar (or carbohydrates) and alcohol is turned by the body into glucose. Glucose is the fuel our bodies run on. If you don't need glucose the excess is turned into fat. So, too much fat, carbohydrate or alcohol can all lead to fat gain and weight gain. So it isn't just fat that makes you fat. Nor is it any old fat that makes you fat.

As far as your body is concerned there's a world of difference between, for example, 100 calories of saturated fat from meat and 100 calories of essential fat from seeds. Saturated fat can only be burned for energy or stored as body fat. Essential fats, on the other hand, are used by the brain, the nerves, the arteries and the skin as well as for balancing hormones and boosting immunity. Only if there's any left over does the body burn it or store it. So you are much more likely to gain weight eating saturated fat than you are eating the essential, polyunsaturated fats.

Similarly, there are good and bad carbohydrates as far as weight control is concerned. Many 'fast-releasing' carbohydrates, which raise your blood glucose level rapidly, are also much more rapidly turned into fat than other 'slow-releasing' carbohydrates. For example, sugar (sucrose) can be more easily turned into fat than fruit sugar (fructose).

Myth 4: There's Nothing Wrong With Being Overweight

The health risks associated with weighing more than you should accumulate as soon as you are as little as 7lb overweight. These include heart disease, diabetes and certain cancers. Once you are obese, the risk of developing diabetes is very high indeed; one study showed that about 40 per cent of heart disease in women is linked to being overweight, while others connect it to higher risks of breast cancer, arthritis, osteoporosis and other complications.[3] According to Dr Susan Jebb of the Dunn Clinical Nutrition Centre in Cambridge, 'Obesity is a serious medical condition that reduces life expectancy by increasing the risk of many chronic and potentially fatal diseases.'

Tried and Tested

The Sunday Times put two similarly overweight people on two different diets: one on to the Fatburner Diet (approximately 1,500 calories), and another on to the Cambridge Diet (330 calories). The Fatburner volunteer lost *more weight* after six weeks. In a larger trial comparing the Fatburner approach to Unislim – a low-calorie, high-exercise regime, with weekly support meetings – the Fatburner volunteers lost, on average, four times more weight (14lb in three months) than the other dieters. Every single trial by third parties proved highly successful. Besides consistent weight loss, there were many reports of additional benefits, such as: 'increased alertness', 'concentration improved', 'no wobbly feeling', 'never felt hungry', 'easy to stick to', 'extra energy', 'thoroughly detoxified'. In these trials not one person failed to lose weight.

The recommendations in this book, however, go further. While the original Fatburner Diet works, there's now an even better way to stimulate weight loss, and promote your health and energy. It's the equivalent to a 'tune-up' designed to reprogramme your body to burn fat. This takes about 30 days. Once achieved, not only will fatburning become much easier, but your weight will be much more stable and less likely to fluctuate with the odd indulgence. Although the 30-Day Fatburner Diet may involve you eating slightly fewer calories than you are eating now, the major emphasis is on the quality, not the quantity of what you eat. And you certainly won't go hungry.

3

Why Diets Fail

SOME DIETS simply don't work, while others can do more harm than good. Be especially wary of crash diets, very low-calorie diets, high-protein diets and 'no-fat' diets. Food-combining diets are not good news for people with blood sugar problems, although they may help those with digestive problems. Also, watch out for miracle cures, slimming pills and fat blockers. As for calorie-counting, it not only encourages obsessive eating, but the maths is patently wrong.

The Con Behind Calorie-Counting

Consider this simple example. A banana is approximately 100 calories, so if you eat one banana less every day for a year you'd lose 36,500 calories. One pound of body fat is equivalent to around 4,000 calories. That means you'd lose 10lb in the first year, 50lb by the fifth year, 100lb after 10 years and vanish completely after 15 years! All by eating one less banana a day.

The calorie equation for exercise is equally ridiculous. Cycle vigorously for 15 minutes each day and you will lose 10lb in the first year. Quite possibly. But 100lb after 10 years? No chance. However, according to calorie theory, a banana every day undoes all that hard work anyway.

According to Dr Michael Colgan, nutritionist to many Olympic athletes, some athletes burn off over 7,000 calories a day, but eat only 3,500 calories. By calorie theory these athletes should have completely disappeared by now.

An investigation by Dr Appelbaum of people enduring famine conditions in the Warsaw ghetto during the Second World War arrived at the same contradiction.[4] With an average calorie intake of 700–800 calories a day, and a requirement of around 2,500 calories, a deficiency of 1,241,000 calories would have accumulated over two years. The average body has 30lb of fat, representing 120,000 calories, to dispose of. Even if all the fat were lost, what happened to the other million calories?

Why Crash Diets Make You Fat

The calorie theory fails to add up because of a missing link in the equation: metabolism. Metabolism is the process of turning the fuel in food into energy that the body can use – and burning off unwanted fat. People vary considerably in their ability to turn food into energy and to burn fat. Those that don't do it well have a slow metabolism and consequently convert more food into fat. Most obese people have slower rates of metabolism than slim people.

One of the serious problems with crash diets below 1,000 calories a day is that the body sees this reduction in intake of food as a threat and slows down the metabolic rate by as much as 45 per cent.[5] According to Dr John Marks from Cambridge University, 'As weight falls, the metabolic rate always falls too.' In the short term you can lose around 7lb of body fluid and, if you're lucky, an absolute maximum of 2lb of body fat a week, which together could account for as much as 10lb in two or three weeks. But the minute you resume eating what you were before, the fluid returns along with the fat, because your metabolic rate has slowed down, meaning that you now need less food to maintain a stable weight. This 'rebound effect' is good business for mortuaries. A report by the National Institute of Health, using the findings of a 22-centre study called the Multiple Risk Factor Intervention Trial, showed that among people whose weight showed a wide variability over six to seven years there was a higher death rate.[6] It's also good for food-replacement programmes, whose customers try crash dieting on average three times a year.

Consider the story of Michelle and Caroline, two volunteers for *The Sunday Times Magazine* Tried & Tested diet feature. Michelle was put on the Cambridge Diet, a 330-calories-a-day food replacement. According to Michelle: 'The first three days were torturous but from then on it got worse. Walking down the road required serious will: I was constantly exhausted and couldn't concentrate so that my work suffered badly. Weight loss came slowly – I'd expected miracles after reading the publicity boasts – but in the final week it finally plummeted. My face acquired the desired gaunt look . . . but, unfortunately, my bust rapidly followed suit. I blew up like a balloon when I resumed eating, and seemed to retain gallons of water; conversely, "loose" skin has appeared, creating an under-arm bat-wing effect. When I first stopped the diet, irresistible bingeing took over but after six weeks, with the exercise of limbs and discipline, I've managed to limit the damage to a gain of 5lb.' Michelle lost 10lb in the month and gained 5lb in the weeks that followed – net weight loss 5lb. This is an example of the rebound effect.

Caroline was put on the Fatburner Diet. She also lost 10lb in a month and gained 2lb on holiday after the diet. When asked about her diet she commented: 'One of the hardest – but best – things about it was the insistence on giving up coffee and stimulants. I had caffeine withdrawal headaches for the first few days, but began to feel wonderful after that, alert and fit and thoroughly detoxified, with no more puffy eyes staring back from the bathroom mirror. I regained 2lb while on holiday, but will whittle it off by eating sensibly.'

The bottom line is that the body is intelligent. If you try to starve it, it will turn down your metabolic fire. If you work against its natural design you'll create problems. If you work with its natural design you'll burn unwanted fat easily.

Very Low-Calorie Diets Can Be Dangerous

Food-replacement programmes involving very low-calorie diets are not as effective as the Fatburner approach in the long run. Due to public concern about the safety of such diets, very low-calorie diets must now provide at least 400 calories and 40g of protein per day for women and 500 calories and 50g of protein per day for men. If you greatly limit your calorie intake the body must break down body fat or protein in order to make energy. The objective is to break down fat, but how can you be sure the body is not breaking down muscle tissue or vital organs? By providing a sufficient amount of dietary protein, the loss of body protein is unlikely.

However, these food-replacement programmes fail on two other counts. Firstly, they do not encourage re-education of eating habits, so when participants come off the diet they are more likely to go back to the kinds of foods they were eating before. Secondly, the body sees a very low-calorie diet as starvation and consequently lowers metabolic rate to conserve itself, including fat. Returning to a previously balanced diet, but with a lower metabolic rate, means a high risk for extra weight gain.

The Fibre Fad

The problems with the calorie theory aren't just mathematical. The main drawback with strict calorie control is that you feel hungry. So, how to follow a low-calorie diet without starving? One answer was fibre, largely in the form of wheat bran. This by-product of the refining of wheat flour has been promoted to a princely food, but partly for the wrong reason. Studies using increased quantities of dietary wheat fibre or fibre capsules have not reported effects on weight loss.

To test these approaches we placed 10 people on a 1,000-calorie diet plus high fibre for a period of three months. Four lasted the course, with an average weight loss of 3.25lb. The high drop-out rate is a reflection of the difficulties of sticking to a low-calorie diet for a long period of time. Another study put 10 slimmers on high-fibre tablets that claimed to induce weight loss for a period of three months. Five completed the three months with an average weight loss of 1.5lb. Not very impressive.

However, some special kinds of fibre assist weight loss. Making your diet high in fibre by eating wholefoods – not by adding wheat bran – is definitely good for you. This is explained in Chapter 9.

The Downside of High-Protein Diets

Fifty-eight deaths have been associated, over the past 30 years, with low-calorie, high-protein diets. Too much protein leads to the formation of toxic substances called ketones, especially if a person is not eating enough calories and therefore has to burn protein as fuel. This isn't easy for the body to accomplish, so weight loss can occur, but at a cost. The increased levels of ketones can induce a toxic state called ketosis, which is both unpleasant and harmful and in the long run can be fatal. In addition to this, when you consume above 80g of protein a day, which is equivalent to bacon and eggs for breakfast and a steak for dinner, you start to increase your risk of osteoporosis.[7] This is because protein is made of amino acids, which have to be neutralised by the body through the release of calcium, an alkaline mineral, from the bones.

Low-Fat Diets Are Not Good For You

Nowadays, one of the most popular diets is a very low-fat diet. There are two potential problems with this approach. Firstly, most low-fat diets are high in carbohydrates. In other words, sugar and refined foods replace fatty foods. This encourages blood sugar problems which, in turn, makes it harder to maintain weight control. For this reason, very low-fat, high-carbohydrate diets can often cause fatigue, mood swings and sugar cravings.

However, a more serious aspect of low-fat diets is the exclusion of sufficient essential fats. We all need two kinds of essential fats, called omega-3 and omega-6 fats. Without these, the body simply can't function properly. In her book, *Beyond Pritikin*,[8] Ann Louise Gittlemann, former Director of Nutrition at the Pritikin Longevity Center, noted all kinds of symptoms in people placed on low-fat diets: low energy, fatigue, allergy, yeast problems, mood swings, and dry skin, hair and nails that she believed were due to the lack of essential fatty acids. Dr Robert Atkins of the Atkins Center for Complementary Medicine in New York, says, 'While Americans have been eating less and less fat, they've actually been getting sicker!'

While most of us should cut back on fat, the real emphasis should be on reducing foods rich in saturated fats and devoid of essential fats (meat and dairy produce), and instead eating foods rich in essential fats (seeds, their oils and fish). These essential fats are destroyed by heating and processing food, so frying is definitely out.

What's Wrong With Food Combining?

A number of food-combining diets abound, based on the principles of Dr Hay, a physician who wrote in the 1930s. He emphasised eating wholefoods, fruit and vegetables; he also advocated eating fruit at different times than other foods since, if trapped in the stomach after food such as steak, for example, fruit can ferment. So far so good.

He also recommended not combining carbohydrate-rich foods with protein-rich foods. So, for example, eating fish with

rice or chicken with potatoes is out. The only study I've seen
recommending overweight or obese people to 'food combine',
i.e. not to combine concentrated protein with concentrated
carbohydrate, showed a 3.5 per cent average body weight
change over 12 weeks. Although subjects in this trial were not
advised to eat less or change the kind of food they ate, there was
no measure to indicate whether this weight loss was solely
because of food combining or changes in the quantity or quality
of food.[9]

It is now known, however, that combining protein with
carbohydrate slows down the release of sugars from food to the
bloodstream, helps stabilise blood sugar levels and thus helps
control weight (see Chapter 5). With estimates that a majority
of overweight people have blood sugar problems, it would
seem that combining protein with carbohydrate would be
better rather than worse for you. Nature does this with beans,
lentils, nuts and seeds, all of which contain significant amounts
of both protein and carbohydrate. So fish with rice is in, not
out.

Dr Hay's approach, if followed strictly, is probably best for
those with digestive problems and worst for those with blood-
sugar problems. I remain to be convinced that the benefits
reported by those on food-combining diets aren't largely the
result of changes in the kinds of foods eaten, rather than their
non-combination.

Those Magic Slimming Pills

Every year a new pill or potion claims to do it all for you. Starch
blockers, fat blockers, appetite suppressants, slimming pills –
avoid all these at all costs. You can't cheat the body without
paying a price.

Starch blockers inhibit the digestion of carbohydrate. If you
can't digest it, you can't gain weight. However, undigested
carbohydrate in the digestive tract is bad news. It feeds the

wrong kind of bugs, causing bacterial and yeast infections, as well as terrible gas.

Much touted as an answer to weight loss is a supplement called chitosan, sometimes called the fat attractor, which inhibits the digestion of fat. It works because it has a positive charge and attracts fats, which have a negative charge. Once bound together with chitosan the fat is less likely to be absorbed, and passes through the body. Unfortunately, chitosan doesn't know the difference between good fats and bad fats. Since the essential fats are probably the most commonly deficient nutrient in the Western world the last thing you want is to swallow something that stops you using the little you have in your diet. Once again, it probably isn't a good idea to have undigested fat in your digestive tract.

Drug companies are also cashing in on the weight-loss market with drugs that stop you digesting fat. Once again, these are bad news, since they also inhibit the absorption of the essential fats.

Some slimming drugs are basically stimulants that suppress appetite and wire you up, inducing anxiety and hyperactivity. Similarly, drinking 15 cups of coffee a day would also work in the short term. In the not so long term, stimulants mess up your body's metabolism as well as your physical, mental and emotional health.

4

Are You Overweight or Underlean?

BEING OVERWEIGHT is not so much the problem as being underlean. Your body is made of both fat tissue and lean tissue (such as muscle). Having more fat than lean tissue increases your health risk, so your body fat percentage is more important than your weight.

Ideally, no more than 15 per cent of a man's body or 22 per cent of a woman's body should be fat. Yet, in the Western world, the average man has a body fat percentage of a little over 20, and the average woman's is above 30.

Your body fat percentage is a little harder to measure than your weight. (With a little patience and a tape measure, you can work it out roughly using the formula on page 194.) Some gyms calculate it by taking body measurements with callipers or with a piece of equipment assessing your electrical resistance. Since fat doesn't conduct electricity, the less 'electric' you are the more fat you have. Some gyms can electronically measure your body fat in this way.

Obesity is Widespread

The next best measurement to know is your Body Mass Index (BMI). To work this out all you need to know is your weight and your height, then look on the chart opposite. (Another chart in

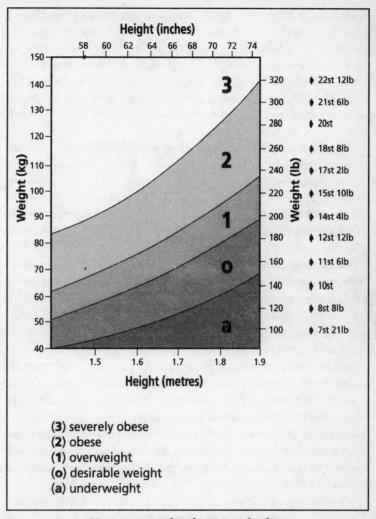

(3) severely obese
(2) obese
(1) overweight
(o) desirable weight
(a) underweight

Know your body mass index

Appendix 1 shows the ideal weight range for each height.) If your BMI is between 25 and 30 (class 1) then you are technically overweight. If your BMI is 30 (class 2 or 3) or above, you are technically obese. If you are overweight or obese you are not alone. Numbers doubled in the 80s and continue to grow at the same alarming rate in the 90s; in some parts of the United States as many as 50 per cent of women are obese. By the end of this book you'll understand why.

If you fall into class 1, 2 or 3, then your risk for weight-related diseases, including diabetes, is much higher. Weight-related diseases account for over 5 per cent of total UK healthcare costs, about as much as the nation's bill for cancer therapy. Being an ideal weight allows you to save resources, maintain your health and have less risk of developing life-threatening and debilitating diseases.

Statistics show that, if you're over 50, it may be better to be a little heavier.[10] A BMI below 23, as well as having a BMI above 28, has been associated with an increased death rate.

A Pound of Fat

Go to the butcher and ask for a pound of fat. It's about the size of this book. In reality, the most you can lose is 1–1.5lb of fat in a week. That means if you're 25lb overweight it's going to take you at least 20 weeks to lose the excess.

The best fuel for the body is carbohydrate. The ultimate aim of the body is to turn carbohydrate into glucose, which then enters the bloodstream. From there the glucose can be delivered to body cells. Any excess glucose is first put into short-term storage as 'glycogen', which is stored in the liver and in muscles. If glycogen stores are full, glucose can be converted into fat and laid down for long-term storage.

Conversely, when you run out of glucose the body breaks glycogen down into glucose. When glycogen stores are used up the body burns fat.

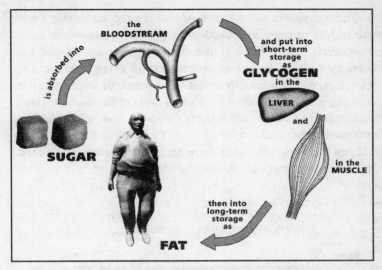

How the body stores energy as fat

If your blood glucose level is fine and your glycogen stores are full, the fat you eat as fat is stored by the body. If you eat carbohydrate your body digests this down to glucose. If your blood glucose level is fine, the liver soaks up this glucose like a sponge and converts it to glycogen, but if your glycogen stores are full, it is converted to fat.

Rapid Weight Loss is Mainly Water

Each unit of glucose your body puts into storage as glycogen is bound together with three units of water. So, if you run out of glucose and start burning glycogen, you lose water. This is how you can develop short-term, rapid weight loss on a very low-calorie diet, for example below 1,000 calories a day. Of course, when you start eating enough for your energy needs again, the glycogen and water stores are replenished and the weight returns.

The measure of a diet that burns fat is a regular weekly loss of around 1lb rather than a sudden weight loss in two weeks. In the two charts below, the top one shows the average weight loss, week by week, of a group of nine dieters on a regular low-calorie diet. In the first week 3lb is lost, in the second 2lb. Things are looking good – a total of 5lb in two weeks. But most of this is water. By the fourth week there's no loss and, presumably as willpower wanes, the volunteers start eating what they need for energy, restoring glycogen and, with that, the water returns. The verdict – an average of 2lb lost in 12 weeks.

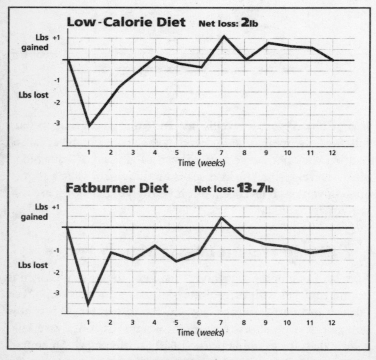

Weight loss on a low-calorie diet versus Fatburner Diet[11]

In the bottom graph, which shows the results of seven Fatburner dieters, once again, there's a sudden weight loss in the first week, but then weight loss settles in at an average of a pound a week, with an average weight loss of 13.7lb per person after 12 weeks. This pattern of weight loss indicates fat being burned.

By changing both the amount and type of fat, protein and carbohydrate in your diet, as well as including certain key vitamins and minerals, you too can burn fat.

PART 2

Your Weight is a Burning Issue

The key to weight control is to keep your blood glucose level even. Excess glucose turns into fat. A lack of glucose leaves you feeling lethargic.
Many factors influence your glucose balance:

- **your sugar and carbohydrate intake**
- **your stress and stimulant load**
- **food combining**
- **the quantity and type of fat you eat**
- **the fibre in your food**
- **vitamins and minerals**
- **hormone imbalances**
- **exercise**

Part 2 explains the nuts and bolts behind the Fatburner Diet, which takes each of these influencing factors and pieces them together to produce a truly revolutionary approach to weight loss.

5

Sugar Makes You Fat

IT IS NO COINCIDENCE that the greatest health risk of being overweight is developing diabetes. What is the link between diabetes and weight control? The answer is sugar. Sugar is bad for you, and it makes you fat.

Sugar comes in many forms and disguises. Most of the sucrose – white or brown sugar – we eat is hidden in convenience foods, snacks and sweets. Maltose is another form of sugar, especially high in refined grains such as white bread or white rice. Glucose, sometimes called dextrose, is added to drinks and cereals, and is also high in certain fruits such as raisins and bananas. Some common breakfast cereals contain every single one of these 'fast-releasing' sugars. They are called fast-releasing because eating them makes your blood glucose level rocket. They need little, if any digestion, and so are rapidly turned into glucose, the primary fuel of the body.

All of these sugars are technically called carbohydrates but the body reacts to these high-sugar foods very differently than it does to other kinds of carbohydrates, such as the complex carbohydrates found in wholegrains, beans, nuts and vegetables. These carbohydrates gradually break down as we digest them, releasing their sugar content slowly into the bloodstream. They are therefore classified as 'slow-releasing' sugars. So too are most fruits, which are rich in fructose, a simple sugar that doesn't really require digestion. Although it can enter the bloodstream quickly, it cannot be used by the body until it has been turned into glucose, a job done primarily by the liver. This slows down its conversion into glucose, making most fruits 'slow-releasing'.

Why Sugar Makes You Fat

Sugar is absorbed into the bloodstream so that it can be delivered to cells such as those in the brain and muscles, as a source of energy-giving fuel. Unfortunately glucose, a high-octane fuel, is dangerous. If levels in the blood are too high it creates damage leading to nerve, eye, kidney and artery damage in diabetics. For this reason, the second your blood sugar level rises too high the body moves quickly to expel the sugar from the bloodstream and, if you don't need it for energy, it dumps it into storage as fat. This is why controlling your blood sugar levels is absolutely crucial if you want to avoid building up fat.

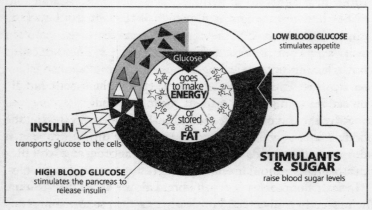

The sugar cycle

The job of moving sugar out of the blood is done by insulin, a hormone produced by the pancreas. The more frequently your blood sugar is raised, the more insulin you produce. The more insulin you produce, the more sugar you dump as fat. Insulin can therefore be thought of as the fat-storing hormone.

A high insulin level encourages not only the conversion of food into fat, but it also inhibits the body's breakdown of previous stores of fat. So, once you're fat you stay fat. Too much insulin is truly a Fatburner's enemy, so, if you are overweight, it's probably your enemy too. According to Professor Gerald Reaven from Stanford University, the majority of obese people and 25 per cent of non-obese people overproduce insulin.[12]

Glucagon, another hormone from the pancreas, is a Fatburner's friend. Imagine this sensitive see-saw of blood glucose levels. You eat carbohydrates and your blood glucose level rises. Insulin is released and it falls. Unless you eat again it's going to stay down, which is what triggers hunger. Too low a blood glucose level then triggers the release of glucagon, a hormone that tells the body to break down fat and burn it for energy, so glucagon is a fatburning hormone. The more glucagon you produce, in relation to insulin, the more you are programming yourself to burn fat.

The chart over the page shows this balancing act between your blood glucose level, insulin and glucagon. If you eat the kinds of foods to keep your blood glucose level in check, the body produces little insulin, so that whenever your energy is low, it releases glucagon to burn some fat. On the other hand, if you eat the wrong kinds of foods, your blood sugar level keeps shooting up, and out pours the insulin and on creeps the fat. So burning fat is very much dependent on eating the right foods to keep your blood sugar levels from rising, in order to avoid the release of large amounts of insulin.

In fact, the more often you stimulate the release of insulin the more insensitive your body becomes to it, so the more you have to produce. This syndrome is called 'insulin resistance'.

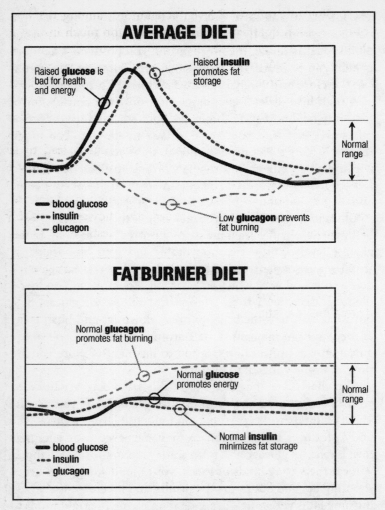

Blood sugar balance

According to Professor Reaven at Stanford, among the non-obese, about a quarter of people produce too much insulin in response to eating carbohydrate and therefore are prone to weight gain; half have a normal insulin response and will therefore only produce too much insulin if they are eating too many fast-releasing sugars; and a quarter have a low insulin response and are therefore less likely to gain weight unless they are substantially overeating. A majority of overweight people produce too much insulin, which can eventually lead to an inability to respond to it properly. But how do you know if you are insulin-resistant or sugar-sensitive? Nutritionists can run blood tests to find out how you respond; your symptoms and your relationship with sugar are, however, a fairly accurate guide. Ask yourself the following questions:

Are you sugar sensitive?	Yes	No
Are you rarely wide awake within 20 minutes of getting up?		
Do you need tea, coffee, a cigarette or something to get you going in the morning?		
Do you really like sweet foods?		
Do you crave bread, cereal, popcorn or pasta most days?		
Do you feel like you 'need' an alcoholic drink most days?		
Are you overweight and unable to shift the extra pounds?		
Do you often have energy slumps during the day or after meals?		
Do you often have mood swings or difficulty concentrating?		

chart continues

	Yes	No
Do you fall asleep in the early evening or need naps during the day?		
Do you avoid exercise because you haven't got the energy?		
Do you get dizzy or irritable if you go six hours without food?		
Do you often find you over-react to stress?		
Do you often get irritable, angry or aggressive unexpectedly?		
Is your energy now less than it used to be?		
Do you get night sweats or frequent headaches?		
Do you ever lie about how much sweet food you have eaten?		
Do you ever keep a supply of sweet food close to hand?		
Do you ever go out of your way to make sure you have something sweet?		
Do you feel you could never give up bread?		
Do you think of yourself as addicted to sugar, chocolate or biscuits?		

If you answer 'yes' to 10 or more questions there's a very good chance that you are sugar-sensitive, struggling to keep your blood sugar level from going up and down excessively. What then should you – indeed every one of us – be eating to achieve the right balance of insulin and glucagon, a major key to weight control?

Balancing Blood Sugar

To become a Fatburner, stop eating 'fast-releasing' sugar foods and switch to foods with 'slow-releasing' carbohydrates that release their sugar content slowly. But how do you know what is fast- or slow-releasing? The very measure of a food's fast- or slow-releasing effect is linked to the degree to which it raises your blood sugar. This can be worked out on a scale called the glycemic index[13] (or GI for short), which measures the level to which a food raises your blood glucose in relation to the effect glucose has (see below). If a food raises blood sugar level significantly and for an extended period of time, the area beneath the curve made by glucose is great. Conversely, if a food hardly raises blood glucose levels at all, and only does so for a short time, the area under the curve is small. The curve created by

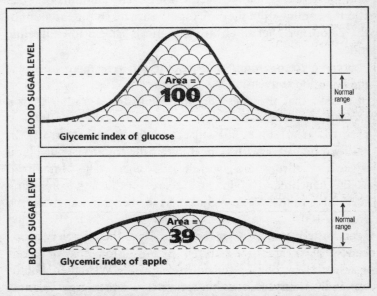

Measuring the glycemic index of a food

glucose, the fastest-releasing sugar, is given a value of 100, and other foods are scored in relation to this. If a food creates a curve with half the area it measures 50. The amount of food tested obviously affects how high the blood sugar level will go. We've used a usual serving size of a food to indicate its relative effect on your blood sugar.

On pages 38 and 39 is a comprehensive chart of the glycemic index of carbohydrate-rich foods based on the amounts you are likely to eat. The higher the score, the more this food raises your blood sugar level.

The Fatburner Diet is principally based on selecting foods with a glycemic index score below 50. However, there are exceptions. Some higher-scoring foods are recommended in the Fatburner Diet, but only when eaten with protein-rich foods that slow down the release of sugar in the blood. Protein-rich foods such as meat and fish are not listed in this chart – they all have a very low glycemic index. The amounts of foods and the combination they are eaten in are taken into account in the Fatburner Diet to ensure that meals have a low glycemic index.

Some glycemic index charts quote different figures because the scientific convention is to measure the effect of an amount of a food that provides 50g of carbohydrates, rather than a serving size. In some cases, such as carrots, the amount you need to eat to obtain 50g is large (800g, or eight carrots). In reality, one carrot with a meal does little to affect your blood sugar level. Also, some glycemic index charts take white bread as the benchmark, giving it a score of 100 and comparing everything to this. We use glucose as the benchmark, giving it a score of 100.

The Glycemic Index of Common Foods

Generally, those foods with a score below 50 are great for your diet, while those with a score above 70 should be avoided or mixed with a low-scoring food. Those with a score between 50 and 70 should be eaten infrequently and only along with a low-scoring food. For example, bananas are quite high, with a score of 62. Oat flakes and skimmed milk are low, with a score of 49 and 32 respectively. A bowl of oat flakes with skimmed milk and half a banana for breakfast would help to keep your blood sugar level on an even keel, while eating cornflakes (scoring 80) with raisins (scoring 64) would be bad news. Keeping track of the scores may seem like hard work to start with but you'll soon get in the habit of it. Parts 3 and 4 explain this in more detail, offering practical suggestions on how to make the right choices.

What makes a food fast- or slow-releasing depends on more than just the type of sugar in the food.[14] The presence of certain kinds of fibre, discussed in Chapter 9, slows down the release of sugars in the food, so that wholefoods are much better for you than refined foods. Therefore it is better to eat brown rice, brown bread or wholewheat pasta than the white stuff. This also means that fresh fruit, which contains the fibre, is better than fruit juices. The presence of protein in a food also lowers its glycemic index, the speed at which it raises your blood sugar. That's one reason why beans and lentils, both high in protein and fibre, have such a low score.

The Best Grains

Some grains are better than others because of the type of carbohydrate, or sugar, they contain. Wheat and corn are high in a fast-releasing sugar called amylopectin, while barley, rye and quinoa are even higher in one called amylose, which is slower-releasing. Most rice has a high GI score because it contains a large proportion of amylopectin. Basmati rice, however, has more amylose and is therefore slower-releasing. Brown basmati is best. (Another reason why lentils and soya are so low on the GI scale is that they contain a substance called an amylase

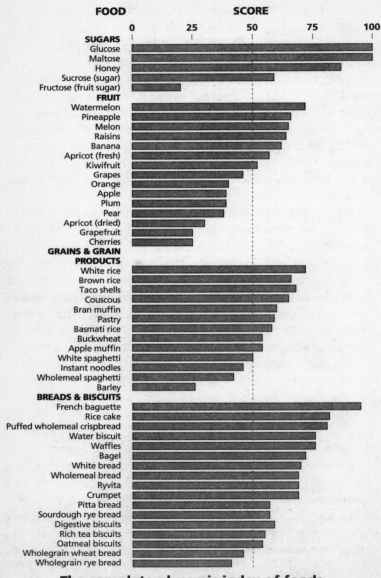

FOOD   **SCORE**

SUGARS
Glucose
Maltose
Honey
Sucrose (sugar)
Fructose (fruit sugar)
FRUIT
Watermelon
Pineapple
Melon
Raisins
Banana
Apricot (fresh)
Kiwifruit
Grapes
Orange
Apple
Plum
Pear
Apricot (dried)
Grapefruit
Cherries
GRAINS & GRAIN PRODUCTS
White rice
Brown rice
Taco shells
Couscous
Bran muffin
Pastry
Basmati rice
Buckwheat
Apple muffin
White spaghetti
Instant noodles
Wholemeal spaghetti
Barley
BREADS & BISCUITS
French baguette
Rice cake
Puffed wholemeal crispbread
Water biscuit
Waffles
Bagel
White bread
Wholemeal bread
Ryvita
Crumpet
Pitta bread
Sourdough rye bread
Digestive biscuits
Rich tea biscuits
Oatmeal biscuits
Wholegrain wheat bread
Wholegrain rye bread

The complete glycemic index of foods

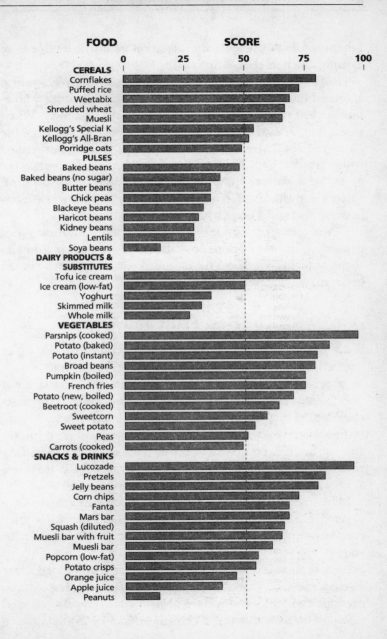

inhibitor which prevents the digestion of amylose, therefore slowing down its release further.)

How a food is processed makes a difference too. When wheat is turned into pasta the GI score is low (especially if it's whole-meal), so it raises your blood glucose relatively slowly. When wheat flour is used to make breads, cakes, biscuits or pastry, the GI score rises. Therefore wholewheat pasta is good, but refined white bread is bad. The best bread is Scandinavian whole rye grain bread, such as pumpernickel, sonnenbrot or volkornbrot. There's a world of difference in the GI – or blood sugar effect – between this and a French baguette.

Of the grains, oats are among the best. The GI of wheat varies depending on what's done to it, but oats are the same in any shape or form. Whole oat flakes, rolled oats or oatmeal, as used in oat cakes, all have a low glycemic effect.[15]

The Best Fruit and Veg

It's a natural assumption that fruit contains fruit sugar, or fructose, which is slow-releasing. However, some fruits – such as grapes, pineapples, watermelon and bananas – contain not only fructose but varying amounts of glucose, which is very fast-releasing, so they need to be eaten with caution. A banana may be fine when you've just climbed a mountain and need instant glucose, but it's certainly not the best daily snack. Half a banana with oats is okay, but oats with chopped apple or pear are better at keeping your blood sugar level from soaring.

Many 'sugar-free' foods use grape juice concentrate as a sweetener. This is akin to using glucose. Some use apple juice concentrate which, being high in fructose, is much better for you.

Almost all vegetables have a negligible effect on blood sugar levels. Vegetables that are worth cutting back on are potatoes, parsnips and swedes which are generally fast-releasing (boiled new potatoes are slower). Although potato crisps may have a lower score, this is because of their high fat content, which is reason enough to avoid them. The same goes for peanuts.

Part 3 gives you a precise eating plan, emphasising the value of these slow-releasing and fatburning carbohydrates.

Health Benefits

Eating this way is not just about losing and controlling weight. Eating slow-releasing carbohydrates improves blood glucose balance and has also been shown to aid the lowering of levels of particularly undesirable fats in the blood.[16] The scenario of having high levels of insulin and disrupted blood glucose control (known as dysglycemia) is associated with a much higher risk of a wide variety of conditions including cardiovascular disease and diabetes, two of the major killer diseases.[17] Eating the Fatburner way not only helps you control your weight, but also helps you avoid the common killer diseases. In summary, the following principles are an essential part of the Fatburner Diet:

- **Avoid sugar in its many disguises.**

- **Avoid foods containing fast-releasing carbohydrates with a high GI score.**

- **Instead, eat foods that contain slow-releasing carbohydrates.**

- **Eat whole, unrefined foods.**

6

The Stress and Stimulant Connection

EATING SUGAR is not the only way to upset your blood sugar levels and your ability to control your weight. Too much stress and too many stimulants can do the same thing.

For emergency situations humans have a 'fifth gear'. In times of stress, the adrenal glands, situated on top of each of the kidneys, release a combination of hormones which help trigger the production of the extra energy. These three hormones help to produce energy by cranking up your metabolism to burn fat. Anything that increases your output of these hormones is called a stimulant. This includes substances in tea, coffee, chocolate, cigarettes, as well as stressful thoughts and a stressful lifestyle. (The stimulant chart on pages 44 and 45 presents a full list of stimulants to avoid.)

The majority of people turn to stimulants for energy because they feel tired all the time. This is the natural consequence of eating the wrong kinds of foods – fast-releasing carbohydrates, devoid of vitamins and minerals. In the short term, stimulants work, as they boost your energy and speed up your metabolism. It's for this reason that taking amphetamine-like slimming pills, or drinking loads of coffee, can produce rapid weight loss. But at what cost?

Are You a Stimulant Addict?

Stimulants are addictive. That's why you need more and more to keep you going. Before long, one cup of coffee and the odd cigarette becomes six more stimulant drinks during the day or 20 cigarettes. By this stage you can't even get going in the morning without a stimulant. Although in the early stages, stimulants like coffee seem to assist weight control, after a while they work just like sugar. They raise your blood glucose level, increasing your insulin, so that the glucose is turned into fat. Regular use of stimulants, far from staving off weight gain, programmes you to put on weight. So too does non-stop stress.

That's why the 30-Day Fatburner Diet advocates cutting back on stimulants. For stimulant addicts this very thought invokes a state of dread. 'Never mind the weight loss, how will I ever get to work without my cup of coffee?' Such a reaction shows just how much we all intuitively understand the body's chemistry. No stimulant – no energy peak. Ironically, we don't realise that the downside, the energy drop, is a result of too many stimulants and fast-releasing sugars.

On the other hand, if you follow the Fatburner Diet, eating slow-releasing energy foods and taking energy-stabilising vitamins and minerals (discussed more fully in Chapter 11), you simply don't need stimulants. Instead, your energy stays even, your blood sugar control improves and you start to burn fat instead of making it. As one Fatburner volunteer said earlier, 'One of the hardest, but best things about it was the insistence on giving up coffee and stimulants.' She also lost 10lb in a month.

STIMULANTS TO AVOID

Coffee contains three stimulants – caffeine, theobromine and theophylline, all of which are addictive. Although caffeine is the strongest, theobromine has a similar effect, although it is present in much smaller amounts. Theophylline is known to disturb normal sleep patterns. Decaffeinated coffee still provides theophylline and theobromine, so it is not exactly stimulant-free. Consumers of large quantities of coffee have a greater risk for a variety of health problems and a higher incidence of birth defects in their children. Coffee stops vital minerals being absorbed. The amount of iron absorbed is reduced to one-third if coffee is drunk with a meal.

Tea is the great British addiction. A strong cup of tea contains as much caffeine as a weak cup of coffee, and it is certainly addictive. Tea also contains tannin, which interferes with the absorption of vital minerals such as iron and zinc. Like coffee, drinking too much tea is also associated with a number of health problems, including an increased risk of stomach ulcers. Particularly addictive is Earl Grey tea which contains bergamot, itself a stimulant.

Sugar is the most common addiction of all because of its effect on energy and mood. The more sweet foods you eat, the greater your taste for sweetness. We all have a natural sweet tooth, which is nature's way of attracting animals to eat fruits. In nature, sweet foods are usually safe to eat, but by refining sugar we've learned how to cheat nature and eat the pure stuff. Nowadays concentrated sugar comes in many disguises – glucose (such as Lucozade), malt, honey, syrups. All help the development of a sweet tooth, as does any food with concentrated sweetness, including grape juice or excessive dried fruit such as raisins, although the sugar in most fruit, fructose, does not have the same effect on the body as glucose, malt or sucrose (normal sugar).

Too much sugar is associated with heart disease, diabetes, tooth decay and obesity. It is addictive because of its effect on energy and mood. Eating concentrated sources of sugar increases your blood sugar level, giving more mental and physical energy, at least in the short term. This is one cause of hyperactivity, both in children and adults. It is most noticeable if you have not eaten sugar for a couple of weeks, then indulge in a sugar binge – see how you feel . . .

Frequent overuse of sugar can lead to glucose intolerance, or an abnormal blood sugar balance. The symptoms may include: irritability, aggressive outbursts, nervousness, depression, crying spells, dizziness, fears and anxiety, confusion, forgetfulness, inability to concentrate, fatigue, insomnia, headaches, palpitations, muscle cramps, excess sweating, digestive problems, allergies, blurred vision, excessive thirst and lack of sex drive. Does this sound like anyone you know? Probably three in every 10 people have a mild form of glucose intolerance.

Chocolate is full of sugar. It also contains cocoa as its major active ingredient, providing significant quantities of the stimulant theobromine, whose action is similar to, although not as strong as, caffeine. Theobromine is also obtained from cocoa drinks, like hot chocolate. Because of the high sugar and stimulant content of chocolate – and its delicious taste – it's easy to become a chocaholic.

Cola and some other fizzy drinks contain 5–7mg of caffeine, roughly a quarter of that found in a weak cup of coffee. In addition, these drinks are often high in sugar and colourings and their net stimulant effect can be considerable. Check the ingredients list and stay away from drinks containing caffeine and chemical additives or colourings.

Alcohol is chemically very similar to sugar, and high in calories. It disturbs normal blood sugar balance and appetite. Enough alcohol suppresses appetite, which means that 'empty' calories are gained from alcohol rather than more nutritious calories from healthy food. Alcohol also destroys or prevents the absorption of many nutrients including vitamin C, B complex, calcium, magnesium and zinc. The best results in this diet are achieved by being more or less alcohol-free – ideally none or no more than three small drinks a week.

Cigarettes also contribute to raised blood sugar levels by acting as mild stimulants to the central nervous system. There is also evidence that smoking is linked to an increase in insulin resistance. In addition to disturbing blood sugar balance, cigarette smoking drains the body of vital nutrients and contributes to numerous other diseases such as cancer and heart disease. So, needless to say, cigarettes are a big no-no.

Alcohol Makes You Fat

Although strictly speaking not a stimulant, alcohol has a pronounced effect on stress, blood sugar control and weight. Alcohol is the most rapidly absorbed sugar, with one-fifth being absorbed directly through the stomach. It takes almost two hours to use up 10g of alcohol, the equivalent of what's in half a pint of beer.

Alcohol can be rapidly turned to fat by the action of insulin. With chronic use it converts into fat rather than glucose or glycogen and is stored in the liver. Alcohol also interferes with the liver's ability to break down amino acids and turn them into glucose when blood sugar levels are too low. So, in this sense, alcohol messes up blood sugar and fat control, leaving a regular drinker more likely to develop the ups and downs of dysglycemia, and to gain weight. When blood sugar levels are too low, the drinker learns that the fastest route to correct the imbalance is to have another drink. With excess alcohol, the excess blood glucose turns to fat. Habitual drinking can damage the liver, leading to even further inability to control both blood sugar levels and weight. Obesity, alcoholism and diabetes are frequent companions.

The Stress Connection

If you think you are suffering from Pre-Millennium Tension you are not alone: seven out of 10 people consider their lifestyle stressful and as we turn the corner into the new millennium it feels as if the whole pace of life has speeded up. Many people wake up in state of anxiety, arrive at work feeling annoyed after commuting, become stressed at work and go home.

Unfortunately, non-stop stress takes its toll on your body's chemistry and makes you more likely, in the short term, to burn fat than store it, stimulating the release of adrenalin and other hormones that initiate the 'fight or flight' response. This prepares the body for action, by releasing sugar stores and raising blood sugar levels to give our muscles and brains a boost of energy. Unlike our ancestors, whose main stresses – such as running up a tree to avoid being eaten for dinner – required a physical response, twentieth-century stress is mainly mental or emotional. The body copes with the excess of blood sugar by releasing yet more hormones to take the glucose out of circulation.

The combination of too much sugar, stimulants and prolonged stress taxes the body and results in an inability to control blood sugar levels, which leads to weight gain and this, if severe enough, can develop into diabetes.

How stressed are you?

The symptoms below suggest adrenal stress overload:

	Yes	No
Hard to get up in the morning		
Tired all the time		
Craving certain foods		
Anger, irritability, aggressiveness		
Mood swings		
Restlessness		
Energy slump during the day		
Regular feelings of weakness		
Apathy		
Depression		
Feeling cold all the time		

In a survey of patients visiting the Institute for Optimum Nutrition, 54 per cent had a high stress rating at their initial assessment. After six months of improved nutrition, substituting sugar and stimulants for slow-releasing carbohydrates, only 28 per cent had a high stress rating. The amazing thing is that balancing your blood sugar not only affects your weight but also has wide-reaching benefits on your health, your mood and your ability to deal with the inevitable challenges of life. When you're stressed even molehills seem like mountains. When your energy is good and your mind is clear, life immediately becomes less stressful. As Fatburner volunteers from *She* magazine said, 'Increased alertness was a significant benefit. By the third day, everybody felt well – alert on rising, and three of us were bounding about full of the joys of spring.' This is just one of the side-effects of the 30-Day Fatburner Diet.

The only way out of a vicious cycle of stress, sugar and stimulants is to reduce or avoid all forms of concentrated sweetness, tea, coffee, alcohol and cigarettes, and start eating foods that help to keep your blood sugar level stable. Breaking these addictions is easier than it sounds and is explained in Part 3. By changing to the right foods, backed up with specific nutritional supplements, most people feel an amazing improvement in energy within 10 days of cutting out stimulants. That's why the Fatburner Diet recommends you to:

- **Avoid regular tea and coffee.**

- **Stop eating chocolate.**

- **Quit smoking.**

- **Avoid regular alcohol and reduce your overall intake to three units a week.**

- **Do what you can to avoid continuously high stress levels.**

7

Food-Combining Facts

CARBOHYDRATES have serious effects on weight control and blood glucose levels, but very few meals, or foods, contain only carbohydrate. The balance with fat and protein in each meal makes a big difference to how much your blood sugar rises and how you are able to burn fat. The aim is not to raise blood sugar levels dramatically, as this triggers the release of high amounts of insulin, which in turn dumps excess sugar as fat.

Barry Sears, author of *Enter the Zone*, first popularised the idea that combining protein-rich foods with slow-releasing carbohydrates further helps to programme you to burn fat. High insulin is bad news and high glucagon is good news for fat-burning, and protein foods tend to invoke small and equal releases of both insulin and glucagon. Carbohydrates, especially fast-releasing carbohydrates such as refined, sweetened foods, invoke a large insulin release, with little or no glucagon response. Eating fat has little direct effect on either insulin or glucagon. The relative effects of each combination is shown overleaf.

With this in mind, Barry Sears placed 63 women with an average body fat percentage of 29 per cent (the ideal is 22 per

Effects of protein, carbohydrate and fat on insulin and glucagon

food eaten	insulin level	glucagon level
carbohydrate	↑↑↑↑↑	no change
protein	↑↑	↑↑
fat	no change	no change
carbohydrate and fat	↑↑↑↑	no change
protein and fat	↑↑	↑↑
high protein and low carbohydrate	↑↑	↑
high carbohydrate and low protein	↑↑↑↑↑↑↑↑	↑

cent) and 28 men with an average body fat percentage of 20 per cent (the ideal is 15 per cent) on a diet which provided slow-release carbohydrates with relatively high amounts of protein and fat (40 per cent carbohydrate, 30 per cent protein, 30 per cent fat) for six weeks. The women lost 6lb in weight, a pound a week. Their body fat percentage dropped from 29 per cent to 26 per cent and their lean mass stayed the same. In other words, they had burned fat.

The men also burned fat, with a drop in percentage body fat from 20 per cent to 17 per cent. They had a 3lb gain in lean body mass (i.e. more muscle), explaining the less spectacular drop in weight of 3lb. In other words, they lost 6lb of fat and gained 3lb of muscle. Since muscle is more metabolically active this meant they had also gained a greater ability to burn fat.

How Much Protein?

Very high-protein diets have proven effective in weight control, partly because they help to slow or prevent the body from turning food into fat, and mainly because they cause fluid loss. However, when you eat too much protein without enough carbohydrate toxic ketones are produced in the blood. The body tries hard to get rid of ketones by urination. With that fluid loss comes temporary weight loss. As the body does not like an excess of protein constituents in the blood without sufficient carbohydrates, insulin is stimulated to turn protein into fat.

While we all need around 40g of protein a day, above 80g, on a long-term basis, increases the risk of osteoporosis and also stresses the kidneys. Also, if a person chooses meat as their main source of protein, then their diet will inevitably become high in saturated fat, which is neither good for your health nor for weight control.

The Fatburner Ratio of Protein and Carbohydrate

On a short-term basis, over 30 to 90 days, increasing your protein intake to 60–75g a day, mainly from fish and vegetarian sources of protein, can help restore blood sugar control[18] and help fatburning. For this reason the Fatburner Diet kicks off by providing a greater proportion of calories from protein (25 per cent) than the average diet (15 per cent) as a means of controlling blood sugar balance and reducing insulin resistance. After 30 to 90 days, to maintain the fatburning effect, the protein percentage drops to 20 per cent of calories. A person with no weight or blood sugar problem would ideally consume 15–20 per cent of calories as protein on a long-term basis. Practical suggestions of how to apply this are provided in clear and simple terms in Part 3.

The perfect balance

	protein	carbohydrate	fat
average diet	15%	45%	40%
Fatburner Diet (first 30–90 days)	25%	50%	25%
Fatburner Diet (maintenance after 90 days)	15–20%	55–60%	25%

Since we all need to eat some protein, some carbohydrate and the right kind of fat, the best combination is to eat reasonably slow-releasing carbohydrates such as oats and rye with foods rich in protein.

The easiest and healthiest way to achieve 60g of protein and 120g of carbohydrate in a day is to divide it evenly between each meal, i.e. 20g of protein and 40g of carbohydrate at breakfast, at lunch and at dinner. Details on the quantity and quality of fats to be eaten are given in Chapter 8.

The simplest way to visualise your meals, as far as lunch and dinner are concerned, is to eat any one of the protein-rich foods shown below, with an equivalent-sized serving of any carbohydrate-rich food, plus two servings of vegetables.

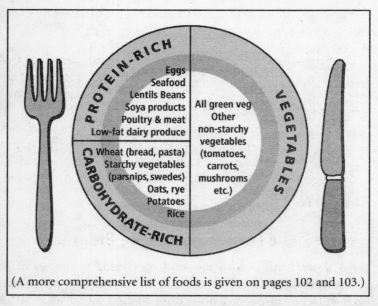

PROTEIN-RICH

Eggs
Seafood
Lentils Beans
Soya products
Poultry & meat
Low-fat dairy produce

CARBOHYDRATE-RICH

Wheat (bread, pasta)
Starchy vegetables
(parsnips, swedes)
Oats, rye
Potatoes
Rice

VEGETABLES

All green veg
Other
non-starchy
vegetables
(tomatoes,
carrots,
mushrooms
etc.)

(A more comprehensive list of foods is given on pages 102 and 103.)

Fatburning food combinations

To maximise fatburning you will probably eat more protein-rich foods in relation to carbohydrate-rich foods than you are used to, as well as more fresh fruit and vegetables. The amount of carbohydrate or protein provided by non-starchy vegetables (such as broccoli, kale, cabbage, peas, spinach or carrots) is small so these can be eaten relatively freely on the Fatburner Diet. Aim for two servings of vegetables with each main meal.

Here are a few examples:

protein	carbohydrate	vegetables
poached salmon . . .	on brown basmati rice . . .	with a green salad
marinated tofu . . .	on wholewheat pasta . . .	steam-fried with vegetables
grilled chicken breast . . .	with boiled new potatoes . . .	with steamed runner beans
cottage cheese . . .	on oat cakes . . .	with broccoli and tomato salad

The Fatburner Diet includes two 'slow-releasing' pieces of fruit as snacks between meals. Their effect on your blood sugar can be slowed down even more by eating a few pumpkin seeds, high in protein, at the same time.

For breakfast you can achieve the right balance and amount of protein and carbohydrate by, for example, eating a cup of oatflakes with some seeds, some chopped fruit and either skimmed milk or soya milk. Detailed menus and recipes are provided in Part 4.

The Food-Combining Enigma

For those familiar with the food-combining principles of Dr Hay this advice may seem unusual. To solve digestive problems, Dr Hay recommended not eating protein along with carbohydrates. This particular part of his dietary theory has received

much criticism in the light of recent research showing the benefit on blood sugar control of combining such foods. While most
of his dietary recommendations have stood the test of time, this
particular aspect is in need of revision, especially for those with
poor blood sugar control and corresponding weight problems.

The key principles behind all the examples given in this
chapter are to:

- **Make sure your meals and snacks provide a
  balance of protein and carbohydrate.**

- **Ensure a daily protein intake (for the first 30 days)
  of 60g.**

8

Good Fats and Bad Fats

THERE IS NO doubt that most people eat too much fat, but some kinds of fat actually improve your ability to burn body fat. So entrenched have we become in fatphobia and the promotion of low-fat diets that the role of essential fats in helping you to burn fat has gone largely unnoticed.

The original idea was that, since 1g of fat gives more calories (9kcals) than 1g of protein or carbohydrate (4kcals), then the quickest way to cut calories was to cut fat. But then we discovered there were essential fats (polyunsaturates) and non-essential fats (saturates). When you eat 100g of saturated fat, all your body can do is burn it for energy or store it as fat. On the other hand, when you eat 100g of the essential polyunsaturated fats from seeds, seed oils or fish, it is used by the brain and nerves, boosts immunity, balances hormones, reduces inflammation and promotes healthy skin. Only if any is left after that will the body use essential fats for energy or store it as fat. In other words, 1 calorie of saturated fat has an entirely different effect on the body in terms of weight control, than 1 calorie of polyunsaturated fat.

Furthermore, certain kinds of polyunsaturated fats help make hormone-like substances called prostaglandins which control metabolism, fatburning and also inflammation. The best kinds of polyunsaturated fats for this are known as the omega-3 essential fats, from flax seeds, pumpkin seeds and fish, especially carnivorous coldwater fish such as mackerel, herring, salmon and tuna. Consuming such foods is very beneficial, while eating meat and dairy produce, both of which are rich in saturated fat, is not so good. For many people, the Fatburner Diet will involve reducing the amount of protein they get from meat and dairy foods – the menus and recipes in Part 4 will help you with this.

There is also an 'in-between' fat, called monounsaturated fat; olive oil is a particularly rich source. While this is nowhere near as good for you as food sources of the omega-3 fats, it is also nowhere near as bad for you as saturated fat. One study found that switching people from saturated to monounsaturated fats helps to stabilise blood sugar levels, improve insulin resistance and control diabetes.[19]

Say No to Saturated Fat

To lose weight, it is definitely desirable to cut down on saturated fat. Nowadays even the average child consumes over 700lb of saturated fat – the equivalent of 1,314 packets of lard between the ages of 6 and 16. Excessive fat is associated with obesity,[20] heart disease, cancer and diabetes and it puts extra stress on the body's metabolism.

Hydrogenated is the 'H' Word

Although essential polyunsaturated fats in their purest form have beneficial qualities, polyunsaturated fats which have been processed, fried or damaged are just as bad for you as saturated fats. If not worse. When the molecules of these essential fats are altered by food processing (called hydrogenation) or frying they can no longer do good in the body and are called trans fats. In addition, frying or heating can make them rancid, or oxidised, which means they can set up a chain reaction of oxidation in the body, damaging body cells. Foods rich in trans fats include:

French fries	potato and corn chips and crisps
hamburgers	biscuits
deep-fried fish burgers	doughnuts
deep-fried chicken nuggets	margarine
confectionery	mayonnaise
chocolate bars	most salad dressings

Many vegetarian processed foods are also high in these hydrogenated fats. Vegetable oils become solid through hydrogenation which is why margarine, a liquid vegetable oil, becomes solid – it's been hydrogenated. Check the labels of foods such as veggieburgers or vegetarian sausages. If they include 'partially hydrogenated vegetable oils' don't buy them. Hydrogenated is the 'H' word.

Saturated fat comes mainly from meat, dairy products, butter and eggs (free-range eggs have lower amounts). These foods are also best avoided on the Fatburner Diet.

HOW MUCH FAT?

All authorities agree that our total fat intake should be less than 30 per cent of total calories, but how do you know the percentage of fat in the food you buy? Here is a simple equation that tells you if packaged food is too high in fat:

Check the label for the number of calories per 100g. Now look at the number of grams of fat per 100g and multiply this figure by 10. Is this more than a third of the number of calories per 100g? If so, it's more than 30 per cent fat.

For example, a yoghurt may provide 60kcals per 100g. The fat content per 100g is 3.5g. Multiply by 10, giving you 35. Divide 35 by 60 (0.58). This means that 58 per cent of the calories in this yoghurt come from fat.

Try this simple formula when you next go shopping.

Say Yes to Omega-3 Fats

To lose weight it is neither necessary nor desirable to avoid the essential omega-3 fats from flax seeds, pumpkin seeds and fish. Most of us are deficient in these anyway, so in practical terms, it is best to eat more fish and seeds and cut down on meat, dairy products and other foods high in saturated fat. The omega-3 fats may even help you to burn fat as they help the body to make the fatburning prostaglandins (hormone-like substances), and hinder the damaging effects of insulin.

The figure below shows how the body can make three kinds of prostaglandins (PG) – PG1, PG2 and PG3. PG1 and PG3 are good for fatburning. PG2 is not.

The omega-3 fats from flax, pumpkin seeds and fish can only make the good PG3, but the omega-6 fats, from sesame, sunflower and pumpkin seeds, can produce either the good PG1 or the bad PG2 (the more insulin you produce the more PG2 you make). On the other hand, the more omega-3 fats a person eats, providing the fatty acid EPA (eicosapentaenoic

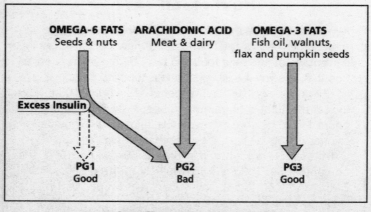

**How insulin and omega-3 fats
influence prostaglandins**

acid), the more they will turn their omega-6 fats into the beneficial, fatburning PG1.

The moral of this story is that you can help your body to burn fat and stay healthy by eating fish and seeds or their oils. The Fatburner Diet specifically includes these essential fats in one of four ways:

- **Breakfast:** A dessertspoon of seeds with your breakfast cereal, yoghurt or Get Up & Go (half pumpkin, half flax is best).

- **Snacks:** A dessertspoon of pumpkin seeds with your fruit snack.

- **Main meals:** A small serving of fish *or* a dessertspoon of pumpkin seeds on salad.

- **Salad dressings:** A dessertspoon of seed oil.

To achieve enough essential fats you need to pick *two* of any of these options each day.

Of course, the fatphobics find this idea hard to swallow. We've been so brainwashed into thinking that fat is bad. In truth, these essential fats clear up dry skin, stimulate your metabolism, boost brain function, protect your heart and strengthen your immune system. What's more, it is now known that the body has a feedback mechanism for fat: fat sensors respond strongly to essential fats and weakly to saturated fats. In other words, your body craves the right kind of fat. If you eat the wrong kind your body isn't satisfied and neither are you, so you eat more. On the other hand, if you eat the right fats every day your craving for fatty foods will diminish.

The amount of fat in the Fatburner Diet, at 25 per cent of calories, is lower than the average diet, which provides about 40 per cent of calories as fat. But the biggest difference is not in the quantity but the quality of fat. Eating in this way means that less than a third of the fat you eat is saturated, compared to two-thirds in the average diet.

The way you cook foods is also important. The best methods are (in order): raw, steaming, boiling, poaching, steam-frying, baking and grilling. Avoid, as much as possible, anything fried, and all deep-fried food.

The Fatburner Diet includes the following principles:

- **Cut your overall fat intake to 25 per cent of calories.**

- **Eat foods high in the essential fats omega-3 and omega-6, with an emphasis on omega-3 fats from fish, flax and pumpkin seeds and their oils.**

- **Avoid foods high in saturated, hydrogenated or processed fats.**

- **Avoid fried, burned or browned food.**

9

The Fibre Factor

IN ADDITION to fast-releasing and slow-releasing carbohydrates, there is another category. Fibre is indigestible carbohydrate, and dietary fibre is made up of all the parts of plants that digestive enzymes cannot break down (although some is digested by bacteria in the colon). It does, however, serve a purpose. When you eat a food high in fibre it tends to slow down the release of sugars in the food which, as far as weight control is concerned, is beneficial.

High-fibre diets are definitely recommended for a variety of general health reasons. People who eat more fibre have a lower risk of bowel cancer, diabetes or diverticular disease, and are unlikely to suffer from constipation. As it is a natural constituent of fruits, vegetables, lentils, beans and wholegrains, there should be no need to add extra fibre if these foods are eaten. Fibre is calorie-free and there is little doubt that a diet high in naturally occurring fibre is more filling. After all, which would you find easier to eat: six squares of chocolate or a pound of carrots?

One of the main reasons why high-fibre foods are more satisfying is that fibre absorbs water, so that they become bulkier in the digestive tract. Every day about 10 litres of digestive juices are released into the digestive tract, so the ability of the food you eat to absorb this water would make a large difference to the bulk of material being digested. Wheat fibre, as in bran, is not very absorbent compared to some vegetable fibres: placed in water it will swell to 10 times its original volume, whereas the fibre from the Japanese plant konjac swells to 100 times its volume.

Soluble and Insoluble Fibre

Although fibre does have an effect on the rate at which glucose is released into the bloodstream, it depends on the type. Intact grains will slow down glucose release the most, whereas ground fibre (such as that in wholemeal bread) has little effect. One of the reasons fruit and vegetable juices are so fast-releasing is that all the fibre has been removed. While insoluble fibre improves digestion by bulking up faecal content and being more effective at reducing constipation, soluble fibre is better for slowing down the release of carbohydrates from food. Many foods contain both types.

Soluble or viscous fibre, such as that in beans, lentils and oats, is particularly effective at slowing down the digestion of food and thereby the blood sugar response. Research suggests that insoluble fibre makes you feel full in the short term, immediately after eating, while soluble fibre reduces appetite nine or more hours later, perhaps by slowing down the release of carbohydrate into the bloodstream, effectively making food more satisfying in the longer term.[21] It's important to eat unprocessed foods such as beans, lentils, seeds and wholegrains, to get the maximum fibre for many reasons, including slowing down the release of sugars into the blood and bulking out your food.

Glucomannan Fibre

Some sources of soluble fibre are used therapeutically to help with digestion, diabetes and weight loss. These include psyllium husks (available from healthfood shops) and konjac fibre (available by mail order, see Useful Addresses on page 209). Of these, konjac fibre, rich in a substance called glucomannan, is the most effective for controlling blood sugar balance by helping to slow down the release of sugars within food into the bloodstream. This means less insulin is required and less fat storage occurs, so glucomannan has significant weight-reducing properties. Of the grain fibres, that in oats comes closest in achieving this, and oats are therefore included in the Fatburner Diet.[22]

Overall, though, glucomannan fibre is undoubtedly the best fibre and has been used in the treatment of weight loss, constipation and diabetes. Two studies, one in Japan[23] and one in the USA,[24] reported an additional 1lb weight loss per week when patients took 3g of glucomannan fibre a day. We decided to put glucomannan fibre to the test by giving 3g a day to 10 overweight people over a three-month period.[25] Nine completed the trial, with an average weight loss of 6.6lb each, with no apparent change to diet or exercise. Our results confirmed the additional benefit of this unique fibre. The main reason for glucomannan's weight-reducing properties is not that it fills you up, but rather that it helps to slow down the release of sugars into the bloodstream.

Due to a quirk in a new food law, glucomannan extracted from konjac fibre is no longer permitted for sale in the UK, although konjac fibre can be purchased. Konjac fibre contains about 60 per cent glucomannan, so a daily intake of 5g would be equivalent to 3g of glucomannan (see Useful Addresses on page 209 for suppliers). For those wanting maximum weight loss I recommend the inclusion of 5g of konjac fibre, taken with a large glass of water, at the start of each main meal.

The Fatburner Diet includes the following principles:

- **Eat whole, unadulterated food, naturally high in fibre.**
- **Eat plenty of food high in soluble fibre (beans, lentils, oats).**
- **Consider supplementing konjac fibre or glucomannan fibre.**

10

Water Retention, Allergies and Bingeing

TWO-THIRDS OF your body is water. By changing the amount of water held in the body you can change your weight rapidly. If you dehydrate the body by not drinking enough water, or by drinking lots of coffee or tea (which cause loss of body fluid), you could lose weight. Another way to lose water is to eat very few calories – as the body uses up your energy stores in the form of glycogen, it loses water too. However this is not the kind of weight you want to lose as it will come piling back on, unless you wish to live your entire life on a very low-calorie diet, guzzling coffee, dehydrating and ageing rapidly. Excess fat – not water – is associated with the problems of obesity.

Drinking plenty of water doesn't lead to weight gain (unless you were seriously dehydrated in the first place). In fact, it's a good idea to drink at least 1 litre of water every day because it helps the body to eliminate toxins released from fatty tissue as you burn it up. It also helps to dilute the blood if it becomes too concentrated in either sugar or protein. (This is why you become thirsty after eating a large dinner or after eating sweets.) Some people have reported tremendous weight loss and health improvements simply by drinking 1–2 litres of water a day.

The body can sometimes retain too much water, creating unnecessary weight gain. This is not a consequence of drinking too much, but results from a loss of the body's ability to control water balance, leading to oedema, or water retention, which can, for example, lead to breast tenderness, experienced by many women before their periods. You can gain as much as 7lb in body weight through excess water retention, and lose it again in 48 hours if you eliminate the cause of your excess fluid retention. If you answer 'yes' to three or more of the questions below, the chances are water retention is part of your weight problem.

- Does your face look puffy, especially around the eyes?
- Does your abdomen, on pressing, feel waterlogged and bloated?
- Do your arms feel puffy rather than pure fat and muscle?
- Do you have dry skin or dandruff?
- Do you ever experience sudden fluctuations in your weight?
- Do you suffer from breast tenderness?
- Are you prone to allergies?

There are three reasons why retention of excess fluid in the body can occur. These are fat deficiency, sugar excess and allergies.

Fat Deficiency

The body holds its water within cells which are encased in a membrane made mainly out of essential fats. If you lack those important essential fats in your diet you lose the ability to maintain the right water balance. On the one hand, your skin dries up and you may get dandruff and become sweaty. On the other hand, your cells get waterlogged and you look puffy and gain weight. The body uses essential fats to make hormone-like substances called prostaglandins which control hormones, and the balance of water, throughout the menstrual cycle. Without these essential fats, the body is more likely to retain excess fluid premenstrually. For these reasons, taking in sufficient essential fats (discussed fully in Chapter 8) can actually help you to lose weight if part of your excess weight is due to water retention.

Sugar Excess

If your body is too full of sugar you'll retain excess fluid too. Wherever it is in the body and in whatever form it comes – glucose, glycogen or fat – every molecule of sugar holds water. If a person is 'sugarlogged' from overeating sugar, then they will retain excess fluid. While it is good to maintain proper glycogen stores, there is no need to have excess fat or excess circulating glucose. Balancing your blood sugar (explained in Chapter 5) helps to prevent excess weight being stored as water.

The Allergy Connection

Many people retain excess body fluid because they're eating something they're allergic to. The word 'allergy' often provokes connotations beyond its original meaning: an allergy to a particular substance simply means an intolerance that causes a reaction in the immune system.

If you are allergic to a particular food, you are likely to crave that food and therefore eat it frequently, as though you were mildly addicted. Through working with a number of allergic and overweight clients, it became clear to me that bingeing, or uncontrolled overeating, often happened only with certain food groups. When clients were instructed to eat as much as they liked of anything other than the suspected allergen (the food provoking an allergic reaction), bingeing often ceased completely. When the allergen was totally avoided clients often lost 3–4lb or even as much as 7lb weight overnight. This sort of short-term weight loss had to be the result of excess fluid retention and nothing to do with fat.

The immune system works with prostaglandins (hormone-like substances) made from essential fats and, if it is responding to an overload of undesirable substances, this can lead to water retention, as well as abdominal bloating. Allergies can be responsible for more pronounced mental and physical symptoms including mood changes, depression, increased appetite, sleepiness after meals, mental fatigue and a host of other minor ailments. Allergies are connected to weight gain in many ways.

One of the physical symptoms of an allergic reaction is a sudden fluctuation in blood sugar level which in turn affects appetite. Could the initial allergic reaction to the food set the scene for increased appetite and hence bingeing? There are no definite answers to this question, but my observations with a number of clients certainly show that sometimes allergies do play a role in overweight problems.

The most common food groups that people are allergic to are: wheat, milk, eggs, yeast, sugar, food additives and nuts. Of all these foods, by far the most common allergy-provoking substances are dairy products and wheat. Almost one-third of people have adverse reactions to one or other of these foods. Cutting back on wheat products, high in gluten, is probably sensible for everyone. Dairy products, which are high in saturated fat, are also best limited or avoided if you prove to be allergic.

A word about alcohol. As well as causing allergies in some people, alcohol irritates the digestive tract in everyone, making it more permeable to undigested food proteins and increasing your chances of an allergic reaction.

By avoiding foods which cause symptoms you will probably find improvements in your health. The Fatburner Diet and supplements (see Chapter 17) will also help to further reduce your allergic potential. After two to three months you may then find that you can tolerate small, infrequent amounts of the allergen. For some people the allergy disappears completely.

Other people have to be careful about certain foods for life. Once you have more than a sneaking suspicion that you are allergic it is often best to see a nutrition consultant, who can test you, advise you what to eat and what to avoid, and help reduce your allergic potential. (If you have ever had a severe or life-threatening allergic reaction I recommend you only do food avoidance/reintroduction allergy tests under the supervision of a suitably qualified practitioner.)

In summary, the Fatburner Diet recommends you to:

- **Find out if you are allergic to something you are eating, and avoid it. It's best to see a nutrition consultant to help you with this.**

- **Drink 1–2 litres of water a day.**

11

Vitamins, Minerals and Metabolism

THE WAY IN which the body uses fat, protein and carbohydrate, as well as water, depends on hundreds of enzymes that,
in turn, depend on the micronutrients: vitamins and minerals.
To tune up your metabolism for fatburning it is essential to
consume optimal amounts of them. For the body to make
insulin, for example, you need zinc and vitamin B6. Insulin's
ability to control blood sugar levels is helped by the mineral
chromium. To turn glucose into energy and not fat you need B
vitamins, magnesium and vitamin C. To burn fat you need all
these, plus the B vitamin biotin.

Turning Glucose into Energy Instead of Fat

The human body is made up of cells. The brain, muscles,
liver, skin, immune system, heart and arteries: all are simply a
collection of cells carrying out work for the body, whether
digesting, moving or thinking. The fuel for all this work is
glucose, derived from carbohydrate foods, so keeping an even
blood sugar level, which provides the fuel reserve for cells, is
the first step in making this energy available.

Within each of our 30 trillion or so cells exist tiny energy
factories called mitochondria which turn glucose into another
chemical, pyruvic acid. This process releases a small amount of

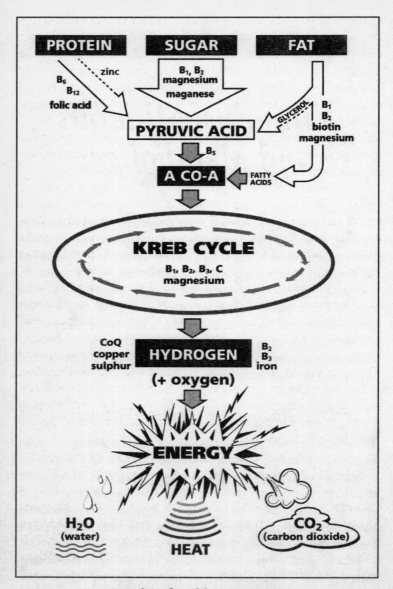

Turning food into energy

energy which can be used by the cell to carry out its work. If this step occurs without sufficient oxygen present, a by-product called lactic acid builds up. That's why your muscles ache the day after the first time you do strenuous exercise using muscles you didn't even know you had. This is, in part, because you've made them work too hard without supplying enough oxygen, causing a build-up of lactic acid. The more you exercise, developing larger muscles, the less strain you put on them, and the more oxygen they can use. Aerobic exercise is all about providing muscle cells with enough oxygen to work properly.

Pyruvic acid then gets turned into acetyl-coenzyme A (AcoA). This substance is perhaps the most vital because, if you're starved of glucose – for example, when a marathon runner 'hits the wall' – you can break down fat or protein to make AcoA, and use this for energy. However this method is rather inefficient so the body prefers to use carbohydrate for fuel.

From this point on, oxygen is needed every step of the way. AcoA enters a series of chemical reactions known as the Krebs cycle (named after its discoverer Ernst Krebs) which separate off hydrogen molecules, which then meet oxygen and – *bang!* – energy is released. Over 90 per cent of all our energy is derived from this final stage. The waste products are carbon dioxide, which we exhale, water, which goes to form urine, and heat. You become hot when exercising, because muscle cells make lots of energy, creating heat, and you puff and pant, to take in oxygen and lose carbon dioxide.

Fatburning Vitamins

Complex carbohydrates and oxygen are only half the story. These chemical reactions are carefully controlled by enzymes, themselves dependent on no less than nine vitamins and six minerals (see previous page). If you have a shortage of these critical catalysts, your energy factories, the mitochondria, will go out of tune. The result is inefficient energy production, a loss of stamina, and highs and lows – or just lows. And whatever your body can't turn into energy easily, it turns into fat. So part of the weight-control equation is to make energy efficiently.

The important vitamins are the B complex vitamins, a family of eight different substances, every one essential for making energy. Glucose cannot be turned into pyruvic acid without B1 and B3 (niacin). AcoA cannot be formed without B1, B2, B3 and, most important of all, B5 (pantothenic acid). The Krebs cycle needs B1, B2 and B3 to do its job properly. Fats and proteins can't be used to make energy without B6, B12, folic acid or biotin.

It used to be thought that a reasonable diet provided sufficient B vitamins. But studies have shown that, in the long term, slight deficiencies gradually result in a depletion of these vitamins in cells. Early warning signs of deficiency are poor skin condition, anxiety, depression, mental confusion, irritability and, most of all, fatigue.

Many people's diets fall short of the requirements for these vital vitamins. A number of surveys have shown that only 10 people eat a diet that provides the Recommended Daily Allowance (RDA) for B6 or folic acid. In one study at the Institute for Optimum Nutrition, a group of 82 volunteers, many of whom already had a 'well-balanced diet' were assessed to calculate their optimal nutritional needs.[26] All 82 were given extra B vitamins in supplement form, often in doses 20 times that of the RDAs. After six months 79 per cent of participants reported a definite improvement in energy, 61 per cent felt physically fitter, and 60 per cent had noticed an improvement in their mental alertness and memory.

Being water soluble and extremely sensitive to heat, B vitamins are easily lost when foods are boiled. The best natural sources are therefore fresh fruit, raw vegetables and wheatgerm. Seeds, nuts and wholegrains contain reasonable amounts, as do meat, fish, eggs and dairy produce. But these levels are reduced when the food is cooked or stored for a long time.

Fatburning Minerals

The minerals iron, calcium, magnesium, chromium and zinc are also vital for making energy. Calcium and magnesium are perhaps the most important, because all muscle cells need an adequate supply to be able to contract and relax. A shortage of magnesium, so common in people who eat little fruit or vegetables, often results in cramps, as muscles are unable to relax. Magnesium is needed in order for more than half of the body's enzymes to work properly[27] and it is vital for the body to use carbohydrates.

Zinc, together with vitamin B6, is needed to make the enzymes that digest food.[28] They are also essential in the production of the hormone insulin, which helps to control blood sugar levels. A lack of zinc also disturbs appetite control and causes a loss of sense of taste or smell, often leading to the overconsumption of meat, cheese and other strong-tasting foods.

The older you are, the less likely it is that you are taking in enough chromium,[29] – an essential mineral that helps stabilise blood sugar levels and hence weight. The average daily intake is below 50mcg, while an optimal intake, certainly for those with weight and blood sugar problems, is around 200mcg. Chromium is found in wholefoods and is therefore higher in wholewheat flour, bread or pasta than refined products. It is also found in beans, nuts and seeds. Asparagus and mushrooms are especially rich in chromium. Since it works with insulin to stabilise your blood sugar level, appetite and weight, the more uneven your blood sugar level the more chromium you use up. Hence, a sugar and stimulant addict eating refined foods is most at risk of deficiency. Flour has 98 per cent of its chromium removed in the refining process – another reason to stay away from refined foods.

Two studies carried out at Bemidji State University in Minnesota have shown that chromium supplementation helps to build muscle and burn fat.[30] Chromium can therefore help to burn fat and, if you're exercising, build muscle. In addition, chromium helps to lower cholesterol and stabilise blood sugar levels, so it is especially helpful for people with a high risk of developing diabetes.[31]

Whether or not you can achieve an optimal intake of chromium from diet alone is debatable. It is therefore wise to take supplements of this fatburning mineral in addition to eating wholefoods. The best forms of chromium are either chromium picolinate or polynicotinate.

The Myth of the Well-Balanced Diet

Even if you eat the kinds of foods that we recommend, you are unlikely to take in the amounts of vitamins and minerals needed to guarantee that your metabolism is as efficient as possible. This may come as a surprise, since we have been led to believe that as long as you eat a well-balanced diet you get all the vitamins and minerals you need. But the sad truth is that this is not correct. Every single survey conducted over the past decade has shown that people who think they eat a well-balanced diet are unlikely to meet all recommended daily intakes of vitamins and minerals.

These recommended intakes, called RDAs, are themselves only set at levels which prevent certain deficiency diseases. They are certainly not optimal levels, which are often many times higher and depend upon an individual's lifestyle, diet, health history and a host of other factors.

Deficiency is Widespread

Why are we so deficient in many nutrients? One serious cause is that we choose the wrong foods. Two-thirds of the average diet comes from refined flour, sugar and fat, all devoid of vitamins and minerals. The refining and processing of food often removes as much as 80 per cent of the nutrients it naturally contains. For example, refining flour removes 98 per cent of chromium and 78 per cent of zinc.[32] However, even wholesome food is not as 'whole' as it used to be. Some oranges contain no vitamin C![33] A 100g serving of wholewheat flour can provide as little as 0.3mg of vitamin B5, a fraction of the optimal intake of 50–100mg. Sometimes, these low levels result from losses due to storage. Food we eat today is obviously not as fresh as that of our jungle-dwelling ancestors.

Modern farming practices also have much to answer for. We acquire our nutrients from plants, or from animals that have eaten plants. Plants make vitamins, provided they take the right elements, including minerals, from soil. Minerals in soil come from rocks being crushed during ice ages, volcanic eruptions or other geological events, so there is a limited supply.

Modern farming methods have allowed us to overfarm the earth, to maximise food production and profit, without putting anything back. To make matters worse chemical fertilisers contain chemicals which bind up minerals like zinc and stop them being absorbed by plants. Pollution, such as acid rain, has the same effect. Since the depletion of many of these minerals does not affect the growth of plants – only their nutritional values – farmers have no financial incentive to remineralise the soil. For these reasons a carrot today is nothing like a carrot eaten by your ancestors, even though it may be the same colour and shape. Food grown by organic methods, avoiding the use of chemical fertilisers and adding minerals back into the soil, consequently have a higher nutrient content.

Hydroxycitric Acid (HCA)

Although not a vitamin, this substance, found in the tamarind plant, could help you lose weight. Originally developed by Hoffman-LaRoche, the pharmaceutical company, HCA has been proven to slow down the production of fat and reduce appetite. HCA has no apparent toxicity or safety concerns. It is extracted from the dried rind of the tamarind (*Garcinia cambogia*) fruit, which has been used as a spice and preservative in the East for hundreds of years, and is thought to be the richest source of HCA.

HCA works by inhibiting ATP-Citrate Lyase, the enzyme that converts sugar into fat. The carbohydrate in a meal is first used to provide fuel and short-term energy stores (glycogen). Any excess is then converted to fat by this enzyme. HCA blocks the ATP-Citrate Lyase. Evidence of HCA's fat-burning properties has been accumulating since 1965.[34] For example, participants in one eight-week, double-blind trial reported an average weight loss of 11.1lb per person, compared to 4.2lb on a dummy pill.

In addition, HCA reduces the synthesis of fat and cholesterol. Animal studies have confirmed this and it may be that HCA has a role to play in helping those with high triglyceride (fat) or blood cholesterol levels. There is also evidence that HCA may enhance the burning of calories and increase energy levels. According to John Sterling, whose company BioCare was among the first to introduce HCA to Britain, 'People are reporting very positive results. HCA doesn't help everybody, but it is helping about 50 per cent of those who've tried it.'

HCA is likely to prove a useful addition to reduced-calorie diets rich in slow-releasing carbohydrates and low in saturated fat. It is widely available as a supplement, often together with chromium.

Fatburning Supplements

I recommend you to supplement your well-balanced diet with fatburning vitamins and minerals to ensure your metabolism is working at peak efficiency. The ideal intake is different for every individual and can be worked out for you by a nutrition consultant (see page 209), but the chart opposite indicates an approximation of the optimal supplement levels for an average person following a well-balanced diet.

	Optimum Daily Intake
Vitamins	
vitamin A	7,500iu
vitamin B1 (thiamine)	75mg
vitamin B2 (riboflavin)	75mg
vitamin B3 (niacin)	100mg
vitamin B5 (pantothenate)	75mg
vitamin B6 (pyridoxine)	100mg
vitamin B12 (cobalamine)	10mcg
folic acid	100mcg
biotin	50mcg
vitamin C	1,000mg
vitamin D	400iu
vitamin E (d-alpha tocopherol)	500iu
Minerals	
calcium	200mg
magnesium	100mg
iron	10mg
zinc	15mg
manganese	5mg
chromium	200mcg
Other	
hydroxycitric acid (HCA)	750mg

These levels are easily supplied by taking one or two supplement formulas, details of which are given on page 209. Most health-food shops can help you to meet these levels in the simplest and least expensive way, choosing from a variety of good brands. Supplements should be taken with food, preferably with breakfast, or spread throughout the day, as we make most energy during the day and hence need a good supply of nutrients. This is why the Fatburner Diet recommends that, every day for at least three months, you:

- **Supplement a high-strength multivitamin and mineral, plus vitamin C.**

- **Supplement additional chromium plus HCA.**

12

Hormones, HRT and the Pill

IT IS NOT AT all uncommon for weight gain to be precipitated by a change in sex hormones. For some women, the pounds pile on during pregnancy, and stay on after the birth. For others, going on or coming off the contraceptive pill or HRT can trigger weight gain. A common time of weight gain for many women occurs during the premenopausal years (usually from 40 onwards) and even more so during the menopause itself, when menstruation ceases. Even more common than weight gain is a change in weight redistribution.

Apples and Pears

Excessive weight on the hips and thighs, resulting in a pear-shaped body, is associated with excess oestrogen, the feminising hormone, while excessive upper body and waist gain is associated with excess androgens, the masculinising hormone.

These hormonal differences are partly genetic and partly a consequence of how we live. Some people have more active adrenal glands, a factor encouraged by a stressful and competitive lifestyle. This leads to the release of more adrenal hormones, such as cortisol and adrenalin, as well as the masculinising hormones – the androgens – which help to build protein and muscle. Hence these 'adrenal-types' tend to be more muscular and have more weight in the top half of their bodies. For such people it is very important not to live off adrenal stimulants (see Chapter 6) and to make sure their fat intake is relatively low. Too much fat, coupled with prolonged stress and a lack of exercise, leads to obesity. In fact, too much of the adrenal hormone cortisol can also lead to excessive amounts of oestrogen (produced in the adrenal glands and fatty tissue, as well as the ovaries), which can lead to lower body weight gain too.

The two key female hormones are oestrogen and progesterone; they are produced mainly in the ovaries and need to be in balance with one another. An increasingly common problem is that a woman produces too much oestrogen in relation to

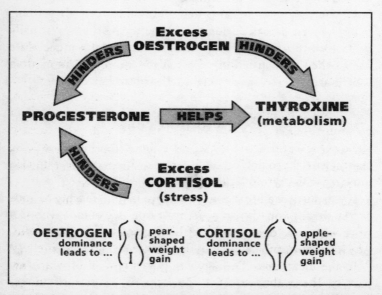

Hormones and their effects on weight distribution

progesterone, usually stemming from a progesterone deficiency, rather than actual excess oestrogen. Progesterone is only produced by the ovaries once the egg has been released at ovulation. If a woman doesn't ovulate – which is increasingly common as a woman approaches the menopause – then progesterone is not produced. After the menopause, progesterone output falls to almost nothing while oestrogen works as the 'feminising' hormone: it helps to lay down fat as storage, especially on the hips and thighs, creating a more curvaceous shape, which is why so many women gain weight in these places after the age of 35. Full details on this subject are given in my book, *Balancing Hormones Naturally* (see page 217).

Men can also suffer from oestrogen dominance. This is most likely to occur when the male hormone, testosterone, is low, as this counteracts the feminising effects of oestrogen. A diet high in meat, dairy and pesticide-sprayed foods can contribute to the development of oestrogen dominance.

Thyroid Problems

The thyroid gland, found in the base of the throat region, controls your rate of metabolism by releasing a hormone called thyroxine which stimulates cells to speed up energy production. Although a relatively small percentage, some people with persistent weight problems have a problem with their thyroid gland. One condition may be that the thyroid is producing insufficient thyroxine, though excessive oestrogen can also interfere with thyroid function.

If you suspect a hormonal imbalance is contributing to your excess weight you should see a nutrition consultant who can work with your doctor to have the necessary tests carried out. Any hormonal imbalances can then be treated appropriately.

In the meantime, the following guidelines, all of which are part of the Fatburner Diet, do help to balance hormones naturally:

- Cut back on saturated fat and hormone residues by eating red meat and dairy products only infrequently.

- Ensure optimal intakes of essential fats from seeds and their oils.

- Eat as much organic produce as possible, to avoid hormone-disrupting chemicals.

- Stay off HRT and the contraceptive pill.

- Avoid prolonged stress and don't live off stimulants.

- Eat plenty of fresh fruit and vegetables and take a high-potency multivitamin.

13

The Best Exercise for Fatburning

UNDOUBTEDLY, a significant reason why there has been a massive increase in the number of overweight people is that we are becoming less active.[35] So many of the luxuries of life simply mean we expend less energy. Cars, remote controls, food processors, home-delivery restaurants, video shops, central heating and elevators are just a few examples of how the conveniences of modern life decrease, bit by bit, our need to expend energy, ultimately leading to the couch potato syndrome.

This is a double-edged sword. Not only does a lower rate of activity lead to fewer calories being burned, but it also interferes with the body's appetite mechanisms, rate of metabolism and ability to keep blood glucose levels stable. In other words, some exercise is essential for the body's chemistry to stay 'in tune'.

According to calorie theory, exercise does little to promote weight loss. After all, running a mile only burns up 300 calories, the equivalent of two slices of toast or a piece of apple pie. But this argument misses three key points.

- **The effects of exercise are accumulative:** Running a mile a day only burns up 300 calories, but if you do that three days a week for a year, that's 22,000 calories, equivalent to a weight loss of 11lb! Also, the amount of calories you burn up depends on how fat and fit you are to start with. The fatter and less fit you are, the more benefit you'll derive from small amounts of exercise.

- **Moderate exercise decreases your appetite:** A degree of physical activity is necessary for appetite mechanisms to work properly. Those who do not exercise have exaggerated appetites and hence the pounds gradually creep on.

- **Exercise boosts your metabolic rate:** The most important reason why exercise is a key to weight loss is its effect on your metabolic rate. According to Professor McArdle,[36] an exercise physiologist at City University, New York, 'Most people can generate metabolic rates that are eight to 10 times above their resting value during sustained cycling, running or swimming. Complementing this increased metabolic rate is the observation that vigorous exercise will raise metabolic rate for up to 15 hours after exercise.'

Exercise Boosts Your Metabolism

Combining diet and exercise is the best way to lose weight. Weight lost through restrictive dieting is often half fat and half lean tissue such as muscle. Since muscle burns up more energy (calories) than fat, less muscle leads to a slower metabolism. Combining the Fatburner Diet with a good exercise programme makes sure you lose fat rather than lean muscle. The best kinds of exercises to help to burn fat efficiently are brisk walking, jogging, cycling, swimming, aerobic dance, stepping, cross-country skiing, circuit-training or any aerobic exercise that is steady, continuous and of a certain intensity.

Such exercises also tone the body, reduce the risk of osteoporosis, increase muscle tissue and reduce one's body fat percentage (high ratios of body fat to lean tissue have been linked to heart disease, diabetes and some cancers). They will strengthen your heart and lungs, reduce your risk of heart disease, help control stress and improve circulation.

Exercise Improves Insulin Sensitivity

According to Vanessa Hebditch of the British Diabetic Association, 'Being overweight reduces insulin sensitivity so the risk of developing diabetes is higher. However, there is proof that exercise increases insulin sensitivity thereby reducing risk.' A 24-year study of nearly 6,000 men found that increased physical activity was linked to a reduction in the risk of diabetes, regardless of the level of obesity.

Exercise is especially important in middle age because as we age, we are less likely to be able to maintain an even blood sugar level.[37] A study of 87,000 women aged between 34 and 59 showed that those taking vigorous exercise at least once a week reduced their risk of diabetes by a third, compared to those who did not exercise.[38] While insulin levels do not necessarily decline with age, sensitivity to insulin does. Physical activity in the middle-aged and the elderly improves insulin sensitivity and therefore helps to stabilise blood sugar levels and weight.[39]

High-intensity exercises, like aerobics, reduce insulin levels and raise glucagon. This means you improve production of good prostaglandins, improve circulation (through the supply of oxygen and nutrients to cells) and you increase your ability to burn fat. For this you need to exercise at 60–80 per cent of your maximum heart rate (see next page).

Anaerobic exercise, such as weights, does not burn fat in the same way or to the same extent. If it is intense enough though, it may release human growth hormone (controlled by good prostaglandins), which builds muscle and burns fat. This effect only occurs at 90 per cent of your maximum heart rate.

Exercise brings so many benefits that you may wonder why you haven't started sooner.

How Much Exercise?

You do not have to be fanatically fit to benefit from exercising. The important thing to remember is to stay within the 'training heart rate zone' for your age. See page 204 to work this out. An overweight, out-of-condition person may reach his or her training heart rate zone by walking just a few hundred yards, whereas a fitter, leaner person may have to walk briskly for at least five minutes to push their pulse up to their training zone. This is why you need to monitor your pulse while exercising to make sure you do not over- or under-exercise, and achieve the best fatburning benefits. As you get fitter and leaner you will find you will have to push harder, i.e. walk faster or add more hill-walking to your programme so that you reach your training zone.

According to surveys, the best longevity benefits occur when you are expending more than 2,000kcals a week. Walking uses up 300kcals an hour, so you'd need to walk for 6 hours a week. Jogging is twice as calorific, so you'd only need to do 3 hours a week. The more overweight you are, the more calories you burn up, so you may only need to do 2 hours.

If you are doing the right kind of exercise you need do as little as 15 minutes a day, both to lose weight and gain shape. That's equivalent to 21 minutes of exercise, five days a week, giving yourself two days off. Alternatively, you may choose to 'double up' and exercise three times a week for 35 minutes each time. It doesn't sound that difficult, does it?

Increasing Your Baseline Activity

One great way to up your general level of exercise is to 'do it the hard way'. Use the stairs instead of the lift. Walk or cycle, instead of driving everywhere. Actively play with the children, or take up a sport. There are many daily activities you can use to develop fitness. Soon, this way of living becomes a habit.

The fat way	The fit way
• Take the lift	• Use the stairs
• Use a trolley when shopping	• Use a hand basket
• Drive to work	• Walk or cycle some of the way
• Drive to the shops	• Walk to the shops
• Spend the night watching TV	• Take up an active hobby
• Ask other people to make you drinks	• Get up and do it yourself (and get them one too!)
• Use power tools for gardening or DIY work	• Use manual tools when it's just as quick
• Go upstairs as little as possible at home	• Run upstairs as often as possible
• Use automatic car washes	• Wash the car yourself
• Stick children in front of the TV	• Actively play with them
• Have business meetings indoors	• Go for a walk where possible

The More You Exercise the Less You Eat

Contrary to popular belief, moderate exercise actually decreases your appetite. According to new evidence on appetite research, both animals and man consistently show decreased appetite with small increases in physical activity. One study looked at an industrial population in West Bengal, India. Those doing sedentary work ate more and consequently weighed more than those doing light work. As the level of work increased from light to heavy, workers ate more, though not relative to their energy output. The result was that the heavier the work, the lighter the worker.

job classification	daily caloric intake (kcal)	body weight (lb)
sedentary	3,300	148
light work	2,600	118
medium work	2,800	114
heavy work	3,400	113
very heavy work	3,600	113

The Fatburner Diet Helps You Burn Fat and Build Muscle

Having the right balance of hormones, especially the fat-storage hormone insulin, helps the body to use protein and, if you're exercising, to turn the protein you eat into muscle. So the Fatburner Diet is a hormone-friendly diet that helps you to build lean body mass (muscle), which in turn, burns fat.

A word of warning for the scale-watchers when you start a committed exercise programme: as you lose fat and gain lean muscle you will lose inches faster than pounds. In the first month you'll look trimmer and feel fitter but you may not weigh that much less. This is because muscle is heavier than fat. Remember, the enemy is not your weight, but having too high a body fat percentage. So check this every month using the chart in Appendix 1, rather than just jumping on the scales. The more lean muscle you gain, the greater your ability to burn fat. That's what counts.

Whatever exercise you choose, you still need to eat the right foods. Generally it's sensible to eat a balanced meal one hour before training, or alternatively a light snack half an hour beforehand. Drink plenty of water while you're exercising, and eat either a balanced snack or a light meal within an hour of finishing a hard workout. Don't get so hungry that you eat the wrong food.

In summary, the Fatburner Diet recommends you to:

- Exercise at least 15 minutes a day, or 35 minutes three times a week.

- Choose aerobic types of exercise that raise your heart rate into the training zone.

- Choose exercise that helps you to build more muscle, which, in turn, burns fat.

PART 3

Get Fatburning Now

14

In a Nutshell

THE FATBURNER DIET is not a gimmick. It represents the state of the art in tuning up your body to burn fat by controlling your blood sugar balance. It's been tried and tested over 20 years of clinical experience. By working with nature – instead of against it – you can lose excess weight and regain health.

The key principles behind the Fatburner Diet (as explained in detail in Part 2) are as follows:

- Eat less, but not so much less that you feel hungry. On average, this means around 1,500 calories a day – though you won't be counting calories on this diet.

- Eat the right ratio of 'slow-releasing' carbohydrates and protein-rich foods in order to achieve better blood sugar balance, stop hunger and reduce your tendency to store fat, while increasing your ability to burn it.

- Eat foods high in fibre, which also help to stabilise blood sugar levels and reduce hunger.

- Reduce stress and intake of stimulants – tea, coffee, chocolate, cigarettes and alcohol – to help even out your blood sugar levels further and improve your energy.

- Reduce your intake of fat, but more importantly, switch from saturated fats found in meat and dairy products to essential fats found in fish, seeds and their oils.

- Increase your intake of vitamins and minerals, both through diet and supplementation, as these assist in turning food into energy, burning off fat and stabilising blood sugar levels.

- Drink at least 1 litre of water a day.

- Become more active and exercise every other day, to burn fat, boost your metabolism and improve blood sugar balance.

Each one of these principles makes a difference. Put them together and amazing things can happen – the sum of the whole is far greater than the sum of the parts. This is the most effective way – the Fatburner way – to reduce your body fat percentage, lose excess weight and gain health without a rebound effect. Follow this for 30 days and you will be a Fatburner, not a fat-storer.

In practice this is extremely simple. In essence, all you have to do is:

- **Eat Fatburner-recommended breakfasts, lunches or dinners, plus two pieces of fresh fruit as snacks.**

- **Take the Fatburner-recommended supplement programme every day.**

- **Do fatburning exercise on a regular basis.**

First you need to get yourself ready.

15

Getting Ready

AS WITH EXERCISE, you need to warm up first. I recommend you take the first week getting ready to start fatburning. Restock your fridge with all the fatburning foods, break your addictions, find the best alternative foods and drinks, locate your nearest suppliers, and accustom yourself to some of the new foods. This is also a great time to try out your exercise options and decide how to fit them into your weekly routine.

Remove Temptations

This is also the time to remove temptations. Start by using up or giving away any AVOID foods (see Chapter 16) from your fridge or larder. This might be a good time to have people round for dinner! Restock your kitchen with the recommended foods and drinks. Do the same at work.

Some of the foods used in these recipes may be new to you. All of them are readily available in either your local healthfood shop, supermarket or greengrocer's. In Chapter 19, you'll find a shopping list, as well as guidance on how to prepare foods that may be new to you. Now that your fridge and larder are empty, fill them up with these recommended foods and drinks.

Setting Your Targets

Most people start diets hoping to lose in a month what they gained in a year. They vow never to eat chocolate again, and to exercise every day. This approach usually ends in failure.

The purpose of the Fatburner Diet is to reprogramme your body to burn fat. While it is specifically designed for you to lose weight, it is equally important to change your body's chemistry so that you become more inclined to burn unwanted fat than to store it. This takes about 30 days. Once this is achieved, losing weight becomes so much easier.

Be Realistic

My advice is to be realistic. Take it one step at a time. Set yourself targets for changing your diet and taking exercise that you know you will achieve. The matter of weight will look after itself. It is far better to take one step towards permanently changing your lifestyle, than to take four steps forward – and four steps back – on an overambitious regime.

After all, we often eat because we are under pressure or stressed. Boredom, frustration, anger and lack of direction all lead to feelings that can be temporarily suppressed with food. Even small dietary changes can be stressful to begin with. It takes time to adjust. So don't worsen your stress by expecting too much from yourself and then failing to meet your targets.

Be Patient

You took years to get fat. Does it really matter if you take months, rather than weeks, to lose it? Our impatience drives us towards the countless 'get slim quick' diets that have been shown, time and time again, not to produce long-term results. It is very hard for the body to lose more than 1.5lb in a week. Anything more rapid is likely to be mainly the short-term loss of fluid. When you eat insufficient carbohydrate for energy production, the body breaks down stores of glycogen, and every lost unit of glycogen loses nearly three corresponding units of water, leading to instant weight loss. But once you increase your carbohydrate intake, the body will restore glycogen stores, plus the water.

What Results Can I Expect?

According to studies on the Fatburner Diet, the average weight loss achieved is 1–1.5lb a week over a 12-week period. That's over 14lb in under three months. It is better not to lose weight faster than this. Weight loss of over 2lb a week will not be all fat loss. The body simply cannot burn off fat that fast. Of course, most of us want to lose 14lb in a week, despite taking a year to gain it!

A sensible target for the first 30 days is to lose 6lb in weight. A weight loss of 1lb a week, maintained over a year, equates to a loss of 50lb. This can be achieved, without any suffering, on the Fatburner Diet.

Don't forget that your body fat percentage is far more important than your weight. Don't just rely on your scales as the only means of checking your progress. As you begin to make more lean muscle you won't lose so much weight, because lean muscle is heavier than the fat you are burning off. But you will lose inches around your waist, since muscle is more compact than fat. Muscle cells are more metabolically active and therefore have the capacity to burn off fat, while fat cells do not. So, as you make more lean muscle, your ability to burn fat increases. Therefore, with the Fatburner approach, you'll be able to consistently lose weight and inches month after month. And you'll also be gaining health and vitality.

The real statistic you want to change is your body fat percentage, though this is not such a straightforward calculation to carry out on a week-to-week basis. (You can do it roughly using the equation in Appendix 1). If you have access to equipment for measuring your body fat percentage – perhaps at your gym – aim to reduce it by 10 per cent each month until you reach the optimal level of not more than 15 per cent for a man and 22 per cent for a woman.

The chart in Appendix 1 shows your ideal weight range for your height. These figures are calculated from life insurance figures. If you're within your ideal range, I recommend that you don't aim to lose more than 4lb a month until you reach your target. If you are above the ideal range, don't target to lose more than 6lb a month.

Setting Your Target

When setting your target, it is good to have long-term and short-term objectives. We call your long-term objective your goal. How you would, ideally, like to be? What do you weigh now? What is your ideal weight? When were you last that weight? What's the most you've ever lost on a diet? Be realistic about your expectations.

Once you've set your long-term goal, which can be filled in on the chart on page 198, work out your short-term, week-by-week target. For example, if you want to lose 15lb, your target after one week would be to weigh 1.5lb less, and so on until the 10th week, when you achieve your goal.

Now you are ready to start fatburning!

16

What to Eat, Limit and Avoid

THE FATBURNER DIET boils down to three basic steps:

- Eat any Fatburner-recommended breakfast, lunch or dinner, plus two pieces of fresh fruit as snacks.

- Take the Fatburner-recommended supplement programme every day.

- Do fatburning exercise on a regular basis.

There are two ways to do this. Either follow the four weeks of sample menus, together with recipes, given in Part 4, or, for the more 'independent' Fatburner or for any time you're eating out, you can devise your own regime using the chart on pages 102 and 103. Simply follow the golden rules and you'll be following the Fatburner Diet.

Whichever way you choose, it's a good idea to follow the week 1 menu. This will provide an indication of quantities, and how to prepare some of the fatburning foods which may be new to you.

Exercise is important for everybody. Combining the Fatburner Diet with a regular exercise programme (at least three times a week) will undoubtedly give you even better results.

It's as simple as that!

Breakfast

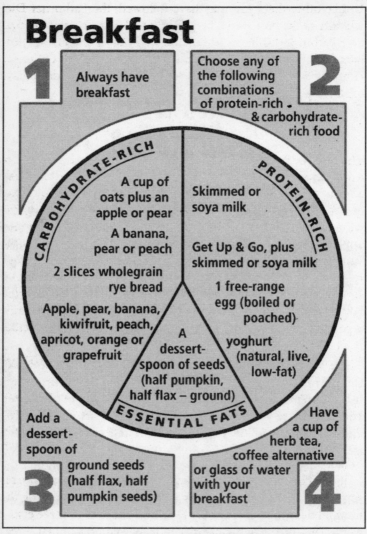

1 Always have breakfast

2 Choose any of the following combinations of protein-rich & carbohydrate-rich food

CARBOHYDRATE-RICH

A cup of oats plus an apple or pear

A banana, pear or peach

2 slices wholegrain rye bread

Apple, pear, banana, kiwifruit, peach, apricot, orange or grapefruit

PROTEIN-RICH

Skimmed or soya milk

Get Up & Go, plus skimmed or soya milk

1 free-range egg (boiled or poached)

yoghurt (natural, live, low-fat)

ESSENTIAL FATS

A dessertspoon of seeds (half pumpkin, half flax – ground)

3 Add a dessertspoon of ground seeds (half flax, half pumpkin seeds)

4 Have a cup of herb tea, coffee alternative or glass of water with your breakfast

The Fatburner Diet: Breakfast

Unlike other diets you may have followed, the Fatburner Diet will not make you starve. According to Hilary Evans, the first ever Fatburner, 'I have never felt hungry on this diet.' She lost over 20lb. You don't have to suffer in order to slim. Quite the contrary. Most people feel more energised and alert within days of starting the Fatburner Diet.

The Ideal Breakfast

The best two breakfasts for fatburning are either: Get Up & Go, a powdered formula that you blend with a piece of fruit and half a pint of either skimmed milk or sugar-free soya milk; or a cup of oatflakes eaten cold like cornflakes or hot as porridge in the winter, with a dessertspoon of ground seeds and a chopped apple, pear or a spoonful of berries when in season. (Some supermarkets sell cans of blackcurrants in apple juice. A spoonful of these on your oats is delicious.) For variety, healthfood stores sell other cereals, for example ryeflakes, that use the Fatburner-friendly grains. However, oatflakes are the best staple cereal and there are many ways of improvising (see the recipes in Part 4).

If you hanker after a piece of bread or toast, find a 100 per cent rye loaf. More and more supermarkets sell these, as do healthfood shops. If you can't find a supplier, why not bake your own? You can also buy whole rye breads in packets with names like sonnenbrot, volkornbrot or pumpernickel. These are so much better for you than regular white or brown bread.

If you choose a yoghurt-based breakfast, check the yoghurt is sugar-free and confirm it really is low-fat yoghurt by using the method described on page 57. Don't eat more than three eggs a week. Two-thirds of the calories in an egg come from fat. Free-range eggs have a greater proportion of essential fats.

Main Meals

1 Choose one serving of a protein-rich and one serving of a carbohydrate-rich food, plus two servings of any of the vegetables. (Exact serving sizes are given overleaf.)

PROTEIN-RICH

Tofu
Tempeh
Soya mince
Cottage cheese
Chicken (no skin)
Turkey (no skin) Quorn
Yoghurt (natural low-fat)
Prawns Mackerel Oysters
Sardines (canned in brine) Cod
Trout Clams Salmon Tuna (canned
in brine) Hummus Skimmed milk Soya
milk Eggs (boiled) Quinoa Baked beans
Kidney beans Blackeye beans Lentils

CARBOHYDRATE-RICH

Oats Brown rice (ideally basmati)
Potato (ideally boiled, new)
Sweet potato Sweetcorn
Corn on the cob Couscous
Pasta (ideally wholemeal)
Wholegrain rye bread
Heavy grain bread
Oat cakes (4)
Parsnip Swede
Broad beans
Beetroot
Pumpkin

3 Vary your diet. If you eat meat and fish, have meat no more than twice a week, fish three times a week and vegetarian meals the rest.

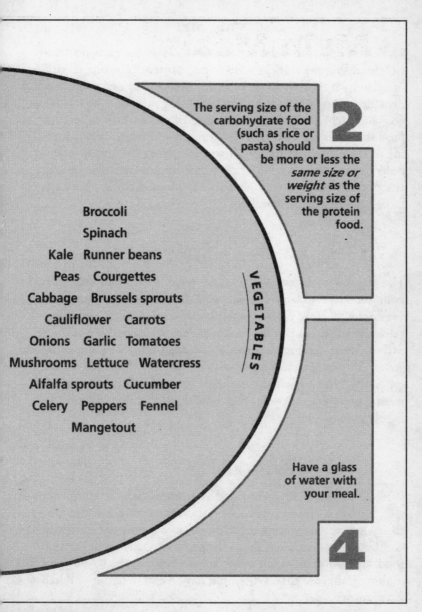

2 The serving size of the carbohydrate food (such as rice or pasta) should be more or less the *same size or weight* as the serving size of the protein food.

Broccoli

Spinach

Kale   Runner beans

Peas   Courgettes

Cabbage   Brussels sprouts

Cauliflower   Carrots

Onions   Garlic   Tomatoes

Mushrooms   Lettuce   Watercress

Alfalfa sprouts   Cucumber

Celery   Peppers   Fennel

Mangetout

VEGETABLES

4 Have a glass of water with your meal.

Main meals

Serving Size

The chart opposite indicates the serving size for each protein-rich food that provides around 15g of protein. The one serving of carbohydrate-rich food, plus the two servings of vegetables provide around 5g, giving a total of 20g of protein, which is the goal for each meal. The serving size of the carbohydrate-rich food should be more or less the same weight or size as the serving of the protein-rich food. If you are eating chicken, which is quite dense and heavy, with rice, which is quite light, the serving size of rice is somewhat larger than the piece of chicken for each to be roughly the same weight.

Vegetables

The vegetables listed in the chart have a minimal effect on your blood sugar and can be eaten freely on this diet. Some vegetables, such as potato, pumpkin and swede, contain faster-releasing sugars so it's best to limit them, or have them as your carbohydrate serving. A carrot a day is good for you, but don't go overboard on parsnips, as they have a high GI score, especially when cooked. The best vegetables to choose are fresh vegetables, organic if possible, eaten raw, steamed or lightly cooked.

Beans and Lentils

While beans and lentils are listed as 'protein-rich', in truth they also contain a significant amount of carbohydrate. For this reason, when you are eating these foods as your source of protein, combine them with *half* the serving size of a carbohydrate-rich food, instead of an equal serving. So, for example, if you were making Dahl (see page 175) you'd have a cup of lentils and half a cup of rice.

How big is a protein serving?

food	weight	serving
tofu	160g	¾ packet
chicken (no skin)	50g	1 very small breast
turkey (no skin)	50g	½ small breast
Quorn	120g	⅓ pack
salmon	55g	1 very small fillet
tuna (canned in brine)	50g	¼ tin
sardines (canned in brine)	75g	⅔ tin
cod	65g	1 very small fillet
trout	65g	½ medium trout
clams	60g	¼ can
prawns	85g	6 large prawns
mackerel	85g	1 medium fillet
oysters	–	15
yoghurt (natural, low-fat)	285g	½ large tub
cottage cheese	120g	½ medium tub
hummus	200g	1 small tub
skimmed milk	440ml	approx. ¾ pint
soya milk	415ml	approx. ¾ pint
eggs (boiled)	–	2 medium eggs
quinoa	125g	1 cup
baked beans	310g	¾ tin
kidney beans	175g	⅖ tin
blackeye beans	175g	⅖ tin
lentils	165g	1.5 cups
Realeat Fishless Fishcakes	170g	2.5 cakes

Vegetarians

Strict vegetarians will need to eat more than usual of tofu, beans, lentils, soya produce and Quorn to achieve the target for protein intake. A serving size of tofu for a main meal is 160g, which is roughly the equivalent of three-quarters of a packet. Part 4 contains a number of recipes and ways to use tofu, which is the vegetarian Fatburner's best friend, together with recipes using a variety of beans and lentils. Many of the recipes containing chicken can be adapted by replacing the chicken with tofu or a tofu steak and the fish can be replaced with a Fishless Fishcake.

Snacks

Many diets eliminate snacks completely as this can be the downfall of many. Those with sugar sensitivity are likely to reach for snack foods to compensate for changes in blood sugar levels and hormonal responses. Most commercial snacks are incredibly high in sugar or fat. A Mars bar, for example, is almost two-thirds sugar with the rest being mainly fat, while even some so-called 'muesli' bars are deceptively unhealthy, made with refined sugar and large quantities of hydrogenated fat.

However, research shows clearly that 'grazing' – eating little and often – is healthier for you than 'gorging' – having one or two big meals in the day.[1] One advantage is that it keeps your blood sugar level even. For this reason the Fatburner Diet recommends that you eat two pieces of fruit as snacks between meals.

The fruit you choose, and what you eat it with, makes a difference. The best fruits are those with a GI score under 50. The chart opposite lists suitable fruits. In terms of quantity, aim for a small apple or pear – some apples are enormous, in which case half would be enough. For smaller fruits, have the equivalent of a small apple filling your hand. You can further slow down the GI score of these fruits by eating them with five almonds or a dessertspoon of pumpkin seeds.

IDEAL SNACK FRUITS

cherries	berries	grapefruit	apples	pears
plums	peaches	oranges	grapes	tangerines

Drinks

The best drink for fatburning is water. Drink at least a litre of water a day. Fruit juices, whether concentrated or fresh, have a relatively high GI because the fibres have been removed. The best is apple juice, although even this should be drunk diluted – half juice, half water, or, even better, two-thirds water, one-third juice.

Alcohol is best kept to a minimum, especially during the first month of the Fatburner Diet. If you can get by without, do so. But if that would be immensely difficult, aim for an absolute maximum of five drinks a week, preferably each one being a small glass of good quality wine.

The best alternatives to tea and coffee are herb teas, rooibosch (red bush) tea, which is good with milk, or Caro Extra, which is a grain-based coffee alternative. (See page 112 for more tips on coming off tea and coffee.)

NEW FOODS

Some excellent fatburning foods, from tofu to quinoa, may be new to you. If they are you can find out how to cook or prepare them and where to buy them in Chapter 19, Shopping for Fatburners.

Grains and Bread

The Fatburner Diet emphasises eating plenty of wholegrains, however this doesn't mean only eating a lot of wheat bread and other wheat products. The best grains for fatburning are rye, barley, oats, quinoa and brown basmati rice. Whole rye bread is better than wholewheat bread. Barley can be cooked like rice and is very tasty in soups and casseroles. So is quinoa, which takes only 13 minutes to cook.

Wholewheat pasta is better than wholewheat bread, as when bread is baked its sugars become more fast-releasing. Buckwheat pasta (Soba noodles) is another alternative. Some of these wholegrains are only available in healthfood shops.

Fats

The right kinds of fats help to programme your body to burn fat. For this reason, the Fatburner Diet recommends that you include essential fats in one of four ways:

- **Breakfast:** A dessertspoon of seeds on your cereal, yoghurt or Get Up & Go (half pumpkin, half flax is best).

- **Snacks:** A dessertspoon of pumpkin seeds with your fruit snack.

- **Main meals:** A small serving of fish *or* a dessertspoon of pumpkin seeds on a salad.

- **Salad dressings:** A dessertspoon of seed oil.

To achieve enough essential fats, you need to *pick two of any of these options* each day. So if you have seeds in your breakfast cereal and seeds with your fruit snack you've had enough for the day. If you have fish for lunch and a salad with seed oil in the evening, there's no need to add seeds to your breakfast as well.

Flax seeds are the best seeds for fatburning, and pumpkin seeds are next best. Flax seeds are, however, so small you don't get much benefit from them unless you grind them. For breakfast I recommend you put equal portions of flax and pumpkin seeds in your now redundant coffee grinder. For snacks, just nibble on a few pumpkin seeds with your piece of fruit. If you have two pieces of fruit as snacks you'll need to consume around half a dessertspoon with each piece. Flax seeds and pumpkin seeds are available in all healthfood shops; pumpkin seeds may also be available in your local supermarket. The dark green pumpkin seeds are the best.

When using seed oils for salad dressings, select either flax seed oil or a blend of oils that gives at least one part of omega-3 fats to one part of omega-6 fats. These seed oils need to be cold-pressed and in a lightproof container. Two good seed oil blends are Essential Balance and Udo's Choice, available in healthfood stores or by mail order (see Useful Addresses on page 209).

What to Limit and Avoid

The trick with any diet is to fill yourself up with the good stuff, so that there's little room left for less desirable foods. Some desirable foods, like oily fish, still need to be limited because although they contain mainly 'good' fats, too much of any fat is bad for you.

Foods and drinks to limit

These foods are best kept within the guidelines below. Some are included in the recipes in specific amounts because they contain important nutrients. Some are high in fat, while others are high in sugar, so do not have more than the recommended amounts.

dried fruit	Choose fresh fruit or soaked dried fruit.
coconut	Can be used in small amounts to flavour dishes.
seeds	Limit to 2 dessertspoons a day, maximum.
nuts (except chestnuts)	Same as seeds (don't have both; seeds are better).
salad dressings	Stick to the measures given in Part 4.
avocados	One a week, maximum.
vegetable oil and butter	Use sparingly, as in the recipes.
tahini (sesame spread)	Use a small amount instead of butter.
fatty fish such as herring, mackerel, tuna, kippers	Three times a week, maximum.
chicken (no skin), game	Twice a week, maximum.
whole milk and yoghurt	Stick to skimmed milk and low-fat yoghurt.
eggs	Three a week, maximum.
alcohol	None to three units a week, maximum.
coffee	Best avoided, except the odd special occasion.
tea	Best avoided. The occasional weak tea is all right.

Foods and drinks to avoid

These foods are high in fat and/or fast-releasing sugar or are devoid of nutrients. They are best strictly avoided. Once you have attained your target weight they may be eaten on rare occasions.

high-fat meats, including beef, pork, lamb, sausages and processed meats

lard, dripping, suet and gravy

deep-fried food

cream, ice cream and high-fat cheeses

high-fat spreads and mayonnaises

all cheeses, except low-fat cottage cheese

rich sauces made with cream, cheese or eggs

all sweets including chocolate

sugar and foods with added sugar

pastries, cakes and biscuits

white bread

snack foods such as crisps

sweetened, fizzy drinks

concentrated juices and 'fruit drinks'

cola drinks

Breaking Your Addictions

I recommend that you greatly reduce your intake of stimulants such as tea, coffee, sugar, chocolate and alcohol. The important thing is to remember you have these as a pick-me-up. The 'up' is an up from a low blood sugar level. If you have no low blood sugar level in the first place you won't need or crave a stimulant. The Fatburner Diet, together with the recommended nutritional supplements listed in the next chapter, are designed to banish those blood sugar lows and to give you more vitality than you'll ever gain from stimulants.

It is not uncommon to feel groggy for the first two or three days after you give up stimulants and your blood sugar levels dip. For this reason, it is best to start eating the Fatburner way and taking the recommended nutritional supplements for a week *before* you wean yourself off stimulants.

Here are some tips to help you break your addictions:

Coffee Some of the effects of coffee were described in Chapter 6, but the effects of small amounts of coffee are even more controversial. As a nutritionist I have seen many people cleared of minor health problems such as tiredness and headaches just by giving up their two or three cups of coffee a day. When you quit, you may get withdrawal symptoms for up to three days, which reflect how addicted you've become. If, after that, you begin to feel perky and your health improves, that's a good indication that you're better off without coffee. The most popular alternatives are Caro Extra, made with roasted barley, chicory and rye, Barleycup, dandelion coffee (Symingtons or Lanes) or herb teas. Check your healthfood shop for new coffee substitutes.

Tea If you're addicted to tea and can't get going without a cuppa, it may be time to stop and see how you feel. The best tasting alternatives are Rooibosch tea (red bush tea) with milk, or herb teas such as Celestial Seasonings Red Zinger, Paradise Tea and the Yogi Teas selection. Drinking very weak tea irregularly is unlikely to be a problem.

Sugar is perhaps a greater addiction than many people realise. Kicking the habit takes time and perseverance. It is best to wean yourself off slowly as your taste buds will accustom themselves to smaller and smaller amounts of sweetness. Stop adding sugar to cereals and eating cereals containing sugar – add fruit instead. When you want something sweet, have a piece of fresh fruit. Get used to diluting fruit juices with water. Gradually decrease your overall intake of sweet foods. Once you're basically sugar-free the odd sweet is no big deal.

Chocolate is full of sugar and cocoa, which contains stimulating substances. The best way to quit the habit is to stop and find good alternatives. You can eat healthy 'sweets' from health-food shops. My favourites are Sunflower, Carriba and Wallaby bars. Also good are Panda Licorice bars, which are sweetened with molasses. Although any of these 'alternatives' are ways to wean yourself off sweets and chocolate, they should be eaten as an occasional treat, not on a daily basis. After a month, you will probably have lost the craving for chocolate. Be aware that many so-called healthy bars are packed with sugar, hydrogenated fat and other not so healthy ingredients. Always check labels.

Cola and some other fizzy drinks are best completely avoided. Have fruit or vegetable juices diluted with an equal amount of water; some chilled fruit teas make a refreshing cold drink. Aqua Libra, Amé and other soft drinks made of natural ingredients with no added sugar are also good alternatives.

Alcohol If you drink regularly it is best to cut out alcohol for two weeks. After that, aim for a target of no more than five glasses of wine or half pints of lager or beer a week.

17

Fatburning Supplements

NUTRITIONAL SUPPLEMENTS are just that – supplements to good nutrition achieved by eating the right foods. There is no question that optimal functioning of your body requires levels of nutrients above those easily achieved by diet alone. Such optimal levels of nutrients can also help reprogramme the body to burn fat. If you want to know more about how vitamins and minerals do this, refer to Chapter 11.

If you have never taken supplements before, you may find many beneficial side-effects. In a survey at the Institute for Optimum Nutrition, after six months on a supplement programme, 79 per cent of people reported improved energy and 61 per cent felt physically fitter, had fewer colds and a better state of health.

The starting point for any supplement programme is a good, all-round multivitamin and mineral supplement, plus 1000mg of vitamin C per day. Check that the multivitamin/mineral that you've chosen meets the amounts shown on page 77. The all-round supplement alone is very unlikely to provide enough vitamin C (1000mg) or enough chromium (200mcg), so these need to be taken as an individual supplement. Another extra is HCA (hydroxycitric acid). The ideal daily amount of HCA is 750mg, taken as a 250mg supplement three times a day.

An ideal supplement programme looks like this:

	breakfast	lunch	dinner
high-strength multivitamin & mineral	as directed	–	–
vitamin C (1000mg)	1	–	–
chromium (200mcg)	1	–	–
HCA (250mg)	1	1	1

Many brands of supplements are now available so it would be impossible to list all the combinations of supplements that would meet these needs. For example, these two supplement programmes fit the bill:

Solgar's VM2000, twice daily
Solgar's C 1000mg, once daily
Solgar's Chromium Polynicotinate 200mcg, once daily
Solgar's Hydroxy Citrate 250mg, three times daily
Solgar products are widely available in healthfood shops.

Higher Nature's Optimum Nutrition Formula three times daily
Higher Nature's Rosehips C 1000mg once daily
Higher Nature's Citrilean, three times daily (HCA plus
  chromium)
Higher Nature products are available by mail-order (see Useful
  Addresses)

If you are definitely sugar-sensitive, or are in the obese category I'd also recommend you add a supplement of vitamin E (400iu) for the first three months. After that, 100iu a day, which is the amount you'll find in a good multivitamin, may suffice. A nutrition consultant can provide a personalised diet and supplement programme – see Useful Addresses.

If you have Get Up & Go for breakfast it already contains 1000mg of vitamin C so there's no need to supplement extra.

Fibre Supplements

Generally speaking, fibre is not something you add to food. It's already in food, unless a food manufacturer has processed it out. The Fatburner Diet is a high-fibre diet, but, as explained in Chapter 9, glucomannan can help you to lose weight by slowing down the release of carbohydrates that you eat.

Taking 3g of glucomannan a day has been proven to assist weight loss. Konjac fibre, which is 60 per cent glucomannan, comes in 500mg capsules, with the recommended intake of nine capsules a day. Take three capsules, with a large glass of water, three times a day just before meals. As it swells to 100 times its volume by absorbing water it is very important to drink a large glass of water whenever you take konjac fibre or glucomannan. Suppliers are given in the list of Useful Addresses on page 209.

When and How

Vitamin and mineral supplements are best taken with food and – if they are involved in energy regulation – during the day. They should also be taken every day. While most people notice the effects after 30 days, it is best to stick to a supplement programme for 90 days to really notice the difference. There are no dangers with taking any of these supplements on a long-term basis, but once you have achieved your desired weight you may wish to stop taking HCA and additional chromium, which are included specifically to help stabilise your blood sugar levels. Once you have attained this they are not so essential on a regular basis. Most decent multivitamin and mineral supplements will provide around 50mcg of chromium, which is enough if you don't have a blood sugar problem and are not trying to lose weight.

18

Fatburning Exercise

THE MAIN THRUST of the Fatburner Diet focuses on the food you eat, but there is no doubt that exercise helps to keep your blood sugar level even (which is the key to weight control) and to burn fat.

To be a Fatburner all you need to do is the equivalent of 15 minutes of exercise a day, or 35 minutes of exercise three times a week. The exercise programme you choose needs to include both aerobic exercise, which burns fat, and toning exercises, which build muscle that burns fat.

Rather than fumbling with the exercises on the first day, take the first week to find an exercise routine that suits you. You may wish to join a gym, buy a workout video or find a friend to exercise with so that you can keep each other motivated. Set yourself a time to do the exercises every day (except on your day off). You may wish to double up exercise sessions and have more days off by exercising every other day.

Aerobic Exercise

This is exercise intense enough to raise your pulse rate into the training heart rate zone (see Appendix 3), but not so intense that you exceed your capacity to produce muscular energy using the oxygen you breathe in. Sprinting, for example, is too intense: it demands more oxygen than is available, so the muscles switch to making energy anaerobically, resulting in a build-up of toxic by-products.

Here's a list of some aerobic exercises to choose from:

walking	aerobics
rambling	dance classes
jogging	cycling
swimming	team sports
circuit-training	video workouts

The golden rules of any exercise programme are:

• **Warm up first:** This is especially important if you are unfit and overweight. It is worth getting advice from a fitness instructor for best results. Contact your local gym.

• **Exercise at a level which keeps you in your training zone for at least 15 minutes:** If you are swimming, for example, don't stop every couple of lengths. It is better to swim more slowly and keep going than to keep stopping to catch your breath. If you are attracted to team sports like tennis, badminton, squash or football the trick is to keep moving. Short bursts of activity won't do you much good.

• **Set yourself a realistic goal and gradually increase it:** If you run or walk around your local park, time how long it takes. In the beginning make it easy to reach your goal. Then increase the speed, the distance or the time. Gradually, week by week, reach for higher goals.

For example, if you are jogging round a park, one circuit might take you five minutes. In the second week do one and a half circuits. In the third week aim for two. How long does it take? Perhaps 11 minutes. Can you cut that to 10? Keep going until you can do three circuits in 15 minutes. Now you're really fatburning.

- **Vary the exercise so that you don't get bored:** For example, go to the gym twice a week, go jogging twice a week and have a long walk at the weekend.

- **Exercise with a friend, at a gym or in classes, for extra motivation:** Make a regular date with a friend to go to the gym or go jogging and, if they can't make it, go anyway.

- **Drink plenty of water before, during and after exercising:** The body is two-thirds water and you lose significant amounts through sweat and breathing. Drink a glass of water for every half an hour of exercise.

- **Cool down when you finish and stretch the muscles you've been exercising:** Depending on which muscles you've been working, stretch them out immediately after exercising. It is best to hold a stretch and count to 20, rather than stretching, then releasing, then stretching again.

- **Keep it up:** The real benefits of exercise are seen after months, not days. Make exercise a part of your daily routine.

Toning Exercises

By toning specific muscle groups you can lose inches as well as pounds. The more muscle you build, the greater your ability to burn fat, since muscle uses up more calories. Some workouts include both aerobic and toning exercises. Alternatively, you could do a mainly aerobic exercise one day and a mainly toning exercise another. The trick for toning exercises is to have good advice. Your local gym is probably the best place or, if you don't have one, find an exercise workout video that suits you.

One of my favourite home exercise routines is called Psychocalisthenics. Developed by Oscar Ichazo of the Arica Institute, it is a unique exercise system consisting of 23 exercises to develop suppleness, strength and stamina. Each exercise has a specific movement sequence and breathing pattern, almost like aerobic yoga with synchronised breathing. In effect, it oxygenates the whole body, leaving you feeling light and energised. As oxygen is our most vital nutrient for metabolism, Psychocalisthenics is highly recommended for weight control. The whole sequence takes less than 20 minutes and is best learned by attending a one-day Psychocalisthenics training course, although you can also learn it from a video. For details on training locations and supporting material see Useful Addresses on page 209. Psychocalisthenics three days a week, plus three good walks, runs or other aerobic exercise, is a highly portable fatburning exercise routine.

19

Shopping for Fatburners

EVERYTHING YOU need for the Fatburner Diet is easily available in the supermarket, greengrocer's and, for a few speciality items, your local healthfood shop.

Some of the ingredients may be new to you so, as well as telling you where to buy them, this chapter gives you some guidance on how to prepare them. Go out and get stocked up for fatburning using the following shopping list. Everything on this list lasts for a week or more. Fresh fruits and vegetables form a large part of what you eat and need to be stocked up on a regular basis. For some of the foods you will have to investigate your local healthfood store. As the demand for these healthy foods grows, more and more of them are becoming widely available – and the prices are going down.

Your Shopping List

From the supermarket

apples, bananas, pears, oranges, raspberries (fresh or frozen), gooseberries or cooking apples, rhubarb, blackcurrants mushrooms, celery, spring onions, avocado, parsley, carrots, bean sprouts, potatoes, peppers, onions, garlic, cucumber, lettuce

rolled oats and oatflakes

wheatgerm

100 per cent rye bread, pumpernickel bread

skimmed milk

very low-fat natural yoghurt

cottage cheese, low-fat quark or fromage frais, half-fat
   cheddar cheese such as Shape

very low-fat mayonnaise

free-range eggs

tofu – plain, smoked and marinated pieces

brown rice

bulgur (cracked wheat)

couscous

wholemeal macaroni

wholemeal flour

chick peas, various dried beans, lentils

dried chestnuts

mixed nuts, cashews, almonds, walnuts (not roasted or salted)

sunflower seeds

raisins, dried apricots

tinned pineapple chunks

tinned tomatoes, tomato purée

tuna fish in brine

sardines in tomato sauce

cod, haddock, mackerel, herring, salmon

olive oil, cold-pressed

cider vinegar

tahini

honey

vanilla essence

herb teas

Aqua Libra

From the healthfood shop

Vecon, Hugli, Morga, Marigold (or another brand of vegetable
  stock)
tamari (alternative to soy sauce)
yeast extract – low salt (Nalex)
wholemeal lasagne and macaroni, and wholemeal or
  buckwheat spaghetti
millet
alfalfa seeds or sprouts
pear and apple spread (sugar-free alternative to jam)
Whole Earth sugar-free jam
Get Up & Go
dandelion coffee (Symingtons)
Barleycup, Caro or Teechino

How to Use New Foods

Some of these foods may be new to you, so here are some guidelines to help you incorporate them into your diet. (They are
included in all sorts of different recipes in Part 4.)

Quinoa is an excellent source of protein and slow-releasing
carbohydrate. It is reputed to be the secret to the strength of the
Aztec empire, who ate it as a staple food. It is a seed-like grain,
which looks much like millet, that you boil like rice, adding to it
three times as much water so that the grain can expand. It takes
only 13 minutes to cook. The flavour is similar to rice and it is
best eaten as an accompaniment to, for example, a steam-fry or
casserole. You could also use it to thicken soup or eat it cold as
part of a salad, much like couscous.

Tofu is second only to quinoa in terms of protein quality, and
again it is an excellent source of both protein and slow-releasing

carbohydrate. Both tofu and quinoa, when eaten with carbo-hydrate-rich foods, slow down the release of their sugars. Tofu is the curd of the soya bean and comes soft (good for desserts or making things 'creamy') or hard (better for steam-fries or main meals). It resembles a bland cheese but absorbs the flavour of any sauce. So, for example, if you were cooking a Chinese steam-fry, flavoured with soya sauce, garlic and ginger, the tofu will take on this flavour and taste delicious. You can buy tofu already flavoured, such as smoked tofu, marinated tofu pieces and braised tofu. These are firmer and more flavourful than plain tofu and make an excellent substitute for meat or chicken in steam-fries, stews and casseroles. You can also add flavour to tofu by marinating it for 20 minutes. You can even make a tofu steak, or include it in sandwiches. Always drain off the liquid in the packet first. I recommend suppliers such as Cauldron Foods, who guarantee non-genetically modified soya.

Tempeh is a high-protein food made from fermented soya beans. It is available from most healthfood shops in various forms – marinated, smoked, plain, even bacon flavoured.

Lentils and beans are excellent and inexpensive foods that are very much underused in traditional British cooking. Both lentils and beans need to be boiled in plenty of water. Lentils, depending on the type, take between 15 and 25 minutes, though beans need to be soaked overnight, then boiled, usually for up to two hours. Tinned beans are presoaked and cooked and come ready to simply heat and serve. Numerous dishes can be made from beans and lentils, including hummus, chilli bean casserole, lentil roast and soups.

Buckwheat pasta is darker in colour than wheat pasta. It belongs to a completely different food family, free of gluten, and is used by the Japanese to make noodles, sometimes called Soba noodles. Healthfood stores sell 100 per cent buckwheat Soba noodles or ones made from a mixture of buckwheat and wheat. It cooks like regular pasta, but it benefits from the water being changed halfway through cooking so that it doesn't stick together so much. You can also buy buckwheat itself and cook it, like rice, for about 15 minutes in boiling water.

Salad ingredients can be used much more imaginatively than most people think. With a few exceptions most vegetables can be eaten raw. Use raw, uncooked and grated beetroot, cabbage, broccoli, courgette and carrot tops as well as peppers, tomatoes, grated carrots, baby sweetcorn and green leafy vegetables such as watercress, rocket, lettuce, chicory, red cabbage and spinach. In addition, you can add marinated tofu pieces, almonds or avocados (not too often) to increase the protein content.

Tahini is a spread made from sesame seeds and their oil. Being high in essential fats, this is a lot better for you and more flavourful than butter. I use tahini on bread and toast, instead of butter, and for a creamier texture and extra flavour I often add some to savoury dishes at the end. Use in moderation, as instructed in the recipes, and keep it refrigerated.

Seeds contain vitamins, minerals, protein, fibre and essential fats. They are therefore a superfood, often wrongly excluded from people's diets because of fatphobia or ignorance of how to use them. Flax seeds (linseed) and pumpkin seeds are the best for the essential omega-3 fats, while sesame and sunflower are the best for the omega-6 fats. A combination of all four, stored in a glass jar in the fridge to minimise oxidation, then ground in a coffee grinder as you need them, makes a great addition to any cereal. Just 2 dessertspoons could provide your daily intake of essential fats plus other key nutrients, including bone-building calcium, magnesium and zinc. Note that cooking with seeds, especially frying them, decreases their value as a source of essential fats as high temperatures destroy their beneficial qualities.

Seed oil blends need to be cold-pressed and preferably organic. They should be stored in a lightproof container and kept refrigerated. The best blends of oils are those that provide a roughly equal proportion of omega-3 and omega-6 fats. This is usually obtained by combining flax seed oil, pumpkin seed oil, sesame oils, sunflower oil or borage oil. Two such oils are Essential Balance, available from Higher Nature (see Useful Addresses on page 209) and Udo's Choice, available from healthfood shops. These are for cold use only, can be added into soups and cereals, to vegetables or used in salad dressings, and should definitely not be used for frying.

20

Monitoring and Maintaining Your Results

WEIGH AND MEASURE yourself at the start of this diet, and again at the end of every week. Always weigh yourself in the morning, before breakfast, without clothes. Continue to monitor your progress week after week. If you have a bad week, notice any effects on your progress, and get back on course. If you reach a 'plateau', don't worry. This can happen. You can encourage weight loss by following the diet more precisely. Soon, you'll find what you need to do to lose weight, and, once you've reached your ultimate goal, what you have to do to stay there.

A Fatburner Progress Report for each of the first four weeks is found in Appendix 2 on page 197. Fill out the report for week 1. You'll need an accurate set of scales and a tape measure. As scales vary, it's best to weigh yourself on the same ones each week. For the measurements, always take the widest part of, for example, your thighs or your hips, and for your thigh measurement take the average of your left and right thigh. Your total inch loss is the sum of all the inches you have lost from measurements of your bust or chest, waist, hips and thighs. (For example, if you've lost 1 inch from each, your total inch loss is 4 inches.) Your target weight is your short-term objective for this week. Your goal weight is your long-term objective.

At the end of each week, ask yourself honestly how well you've stuck to the diet and exercise programme. A space on the Progress Report allows you to rate yourself with a percentage. This will help you to stay on course. If, at the end of the week, you feel your targets are too hard or too easy, you can adjust the rate of progress you're aiming for.

A spare Fatburner Progress Report is also provided – you can copy it for subsequent weeks.

With a Little Help from Your Friends . . .

Let your friends and your family know what you are doing. Show them this book. Maybe they'll want to join in too! It is helpful to persuade a friend to do the diet with you, so that you can give each other support. Encourage your family to support you by being tolerant with the new foods you'll be preparing and not tempting you with forbidden foods. When you're invited to dinner, let your hosts know about the diet. There are plenty of ways of entertaining on this diet.

You may find it extremely helpful to follow the diet with the help of a nutrition consultant, who can help you get started and will work out a personalised vitamin programme for you. He or she can also keep you on track and provide you with moral support and tips on how to deal with any problems you might have along the way. See the section on nutrition consultations in Useful Addresses on page 209.

Breaking the Rules

Very few people follow diets 100 per cent strictly 100 per cent of the time. No doubt you will break the rules on the odd occasion. This is not a disaster. In fact, I recommend that you allow yourself two meals a month when you can eat what you like. This will help you to deal with special occasions and celebrations. Enjoy yourself! You can always limit the quantity you eat, or eat lightly the following day. Obviously, the more you break the rules, the slower your progress will be, but watch out for your addictions. These have a nasty habit of creeping back into your life. They are best avoided, even on special occasions.

The most important thing to do, if you do go off track, is to get yourself back on track the next day. In one experiment, two groups of slimmers were given an identical milkshake to drink. One group was told it was high in calories, the other it was low. Each group were then given an unlimited amount of ice cream. Which group ate the most ice cream? The group who had been told the milkshake was high in calories. This shows the slimmer's mentality: 'If I've broken my diet I might as well go the whole hog.' Don't act like that. If you blow it one day, get back on track the next.

What if the Diet Doesn't Work?

No diet works for everyone, for the simple reason that there are many different causes for being overweight or obese. Some people find it impossible to stick to a diet (although the Fatburner Diet is very easy). Others fail to lose weight despite sticking strictly to a regime. Perhaps there is some other reason why their metabolism isn't working, such as a thyroid problem or oestrogen dominance. In this case it is best to seek professional advice from a qualified nutrition consultant who can investigate your particular problem or perhaps give the necessary support and guidance you need. There are details on how to find a nutrition consultant near you on page 209.

After the First 30 Days

If you have more weight to lose after the first 30 days and you feel good on this diet, then keep going for up to 90 days. An excellent target weight loss for an obese person would be to decrease their body fat percentage by 10 per cent each month, or to lose 18lb in 90 days. The balance of protein, carbohydrate and fat in the Fatburner Diet (25 per cent protein, 50 per cent carbohydrate, 25 per cent fat) helps to reprogramme your body to burn fat. This reprogramming is especially important for people with a degree of insulin resistance who show signs of sugar sensitivity (see the questionnaire on page 33). Sometimes it takes longer than 30 days.

Fatburner Maintenance

Ninety per cent of the principles covered in this book are completely consistent with ongoing good health and weight maintenance, but there are some things you don't need to keep on doing forever.

Once you have shed most of the weight you wanted to lose, feel a whole lot better, and no longer crave sugary foods, then you don't need to keep eating quite so much protein every day. The Fatburner Diet is based on 25 per cent of calories from protein. Now you can reduce this to 15–20 per cent. In practical terms this means less of the protein-rich foods, and more of the carbohydrate-rich foods on your plate. See the charts on pages 102 and 103, and on page 105, but this time aim to eat between half and two-thirds of the protein portions given, and increase the carbohydrate portion one and a half to two times. In other words, eat a little less protein, and more carbohydrate. This also means an adjustment of the recipes to increase the proportion of carbohydrate-rich foods. Everyone is different in the balance of carbohydrate and protein that works for them, so your best guide is your body. Follow your instincts. Eat what works for you.

Supplements for Life

While it's a great idea to carry on supplementing a good high-strength multivitamin and mineral, plus 1000mg of vitamin C, you don't have to take additional chromium (provided there's 40mcg or more in your multivitamin), HCA or fibre supplements forever. You can safely stop these once you've achieved your goal weight. Chromium is particularly helpful at keeping your blood sugar level stable so, if you ever find yourself craving stimulants or sweet things – perhaps when you're under a lot of stress – you may find it helpful to take additional chromium for a few weeks to help keep your blood sugar level even.

Stimulants – Don't Drift Back

One of the most important – and most difficult times – to stay on track is when you're stressed. At such times those old familiar stimulants (tea, coffee, chocolate, cigarettes, sugar) remind you of their existence. Once you've broken your addiction, don't let them creep back, even when you've achieved your weight target. Daily use of any stimulant is a bad sign. The odd cup of weak tea or coffee when eating out or on holiday, or the odd chocolate dessert is no big deal – but don't make a habit of it.

100 Per Cent Health

Losing weight is just the beginning. Why not go all the way and start to incorporate into your diet and lifestyle all the advice given in my books *The Optimum Nutrition Bible*, and its sequel, *100% Health*? Each allows you to deepen your understanding of optimum nutrition, and help you to achieve higher and higher levels of health and vitality.

FATBURNER RESEARCH

You can help with ongoing Fatburner research. If you've completed the diet for four or more weeks, let us know your results by filling in the simple questionnaire on page 203, answering as many questions as you can. Send or fax it to: Fatburner Research, 34 Wadham Road, London SW15 2LR (fax: 0181–874 5003).

PART 4

Fatburning Menus and Recipes

21

Menus

THERE'S NO END to the variety of meals that fit within Fatburner principles. To help you get to grips with the principles and the recommended foods, here is a menu plan for the first four weeks. I recommend you follow it for at least the first week to give you a clear idea of the quantity and balance of foods that meet Fatburner Diet recommendations. Once you are familiar with your new diet and the basic rules, you can use these recipes and your imagination for a feast of fatburning gastronomic delights.

Should you wish to do it your own way, that's fine too. You can swap meals around from one day to another. However, do bear in mind that each day in these menus is well balanced. They are also balanced for fat, providing two measures of the essential fats every day. So, if you make up your own daily menus, make sure you are not getting too much or too little of these essential fats. Don't pick the highest fat recipe and have that every day. Oily fish, for example, occurs in the menus no more than three times a week. So, as you make your own way, it's good to introduce some variation. There's also enough choice here for vegans or vegetarians to follow the Fatburner Diet. Bear in mind that puddings are a treat, and should only be included on days 3 and 7.

WEEK ONE

DAY 1

Breakfast – Porridge
Lunch – Apple and tuna salad with oat cakes
Dinner – Steam-fried vegetables and tofu with brown basmati rice
Snacks – Two pieces of fruit plus nuts/seeds
Drinks – Unlimited water, herb teas, coffee alternatives and diluted juice

DAY 2

Breakfast – Fruit muesli
Lunch – Fatburner sandwich with green salad
Dinner – Grilled pesto chicken with buckwheat and Mediterranean tomato and broccoli salad
Snacks – Two pieces of fruit plus nuts/seeds
Drinks – Unlimited water, herb teas, coffee alternatives and diluted juice

DAY 3

Breakfast – Fruit yoghurt/yoghurt shake
Lunch – Farmhouse soup with oat cakes
Dinner – Pasta Provençale, apricot whisk for dessert
Snacks – Two pieces of fruit plus nuts/seeds
Drinks – Unlimited water, herb teas, coffee alternatives and diluted juice

DAY 4

Breakfast – Porridge
Lunch – Cottage corn salad with pumpkin seed dressing

Dinner – Poached salmon with boiled new potatoes and
   steamed peas
Snacks – Two pieces of fruit plus nuts/seeds
Drinks – Unlimited water, herb teas, coffee alternatives and
   diluted juice

DAY 5

Breakfast – Fruit muesli
Lunch – Fatburner baked potato and rainbow root salad
Dinner – Sweet and sour steam-fry with buckwheat noodles
   and steamed mangetout
Snacks – Two pieces of fruit plus nuts/seeds
Drinks – Unlimited water, herb teas, coffee alternatives and
   diluted juice

DAY 6

Breakfast – Fruit yoghurt/yoghurt shake
Lunch – Nutty three bean salad with green salad
Dinner – Shepherdess pie with steamed spinach
Snacks – Two pieces of fruit plus nuts/seeds
Drinks – Unlimited water, herb teas, coffee alternatives and
   diluted juice

DAY 7

Breakfast – Scrambled egg with rye toast
Lunch – Stuffed mushrooms
Dinner – Thai baked cod with brown basmati rice and
   crunchy Thai salad, dried apricots with cashew cream for
   dessert
Snacks – Two pieces of fruit plus nuts/seeds
Drinks – Unlimited water, herb teas, coffee alternatives and
   diluted juice

WEEK TWO

By now you'll be getting a taste for the Fatburner recipes. Note the ones you like best, and remember you can exchange lunches or dinner from one day with another day. However, keep your choices varied, since some meals are less balanced than others. Weeks 3 and 4 continue to introduce new and delicious recipes.

DAY 1

Breakfast – Porridge
Lunch – Fatburner sandwich with carrot soup
Dinner – Chilli with brown basmati rice and steamed broccoli
Snacks – Two pieces of fruit plus nuts/seeds
Drinks – Unlimited water, herb teas, coffee alternatives and diluted juice

DAY 2

Breakfast – Fruit muesli
Lunch – Energy soup
Dinner – Spicy mackerel with couscous and green salad
Snacks – Two pieces of fruit plus nuts/seeds
Drinks – Unlimited water, herb teas, coffee alternatives and diluted juice

DAY 3

Breakfast – Fruit yoghurt/yoghurt shake
Lunch – Sardines on toast with watercress salad
Dinner – Mushroom pilaf with steamed courgettes, fresh fruit salad for dessert
Snacks – Two pieces of fruit plus nuts/seeds
Drinks – Unlimited water, herb teas, coffee alternatives and diluted juice

DAY 4

Breakfast – Porridge
Lunch – Rice, tuna and bean sprout salad
Dinner – Harissa with roast vegetables with quinoa
Snacks – Two pieces of fruit plus nuts/seeds
Drinks – Unlimited water, herb teas, coffee alternatives and
  diluted juice

DAY 5

Breakfast – Fruit muesli
Lunch – Fatburner baked potato with green salad
Dinner – Dahl with brown basmati rice and steamed broccoli
Snacks – Two pieces of fruit plus nuts/seeds
Drinks – Unlimited water, herb teas, coffee alternatives and
  diluted juice

DAY 6

Breakfast – Fruit yoghurt/yoghurt shake
Lunch – Crunchy tofu salad
Dinner – Spaghetti marinara with steamed runner beans
Snacks – Two pieces of fruit plus nuts/seeds
Drinks – Unlimited water, herb teas, coffee alternatives and
  diluted juice

DAY 7

Breakfast – Boiled egg with rye toast
Lunch – Mexican bean dip and crudités
Dinner – Roast chicken with boiled new potatoes and
  steamed vegetables, rhubarb and blackcurrant pie for
  dessert
Snacks – Two pieces of fruit plus nuts/seeds
Drinks – Unlimited water, herb teas, coffee alternatives and
  diluted juice

WEEK THREE

DAY 1

Breakfast – Porridge
Lunch – Fatburner sandwich and mixed or green salad
Dinner – Chick pea crumble with steamed spinach
Snacks – Two pieces of fruit plus nuts/seeds
Drinks – Unlimited water, herb teas, coffee alternatives and
  diluted juice

DAY 2

Breakfast – Fruit muesli
Lunch – Tofu and avocado dip with crudités and oat cakes
Dinner – Spaghetti bolognese with steamed courgettes
Snacks – Two pieces of fruit plus nuts/seeds
Drinks – Unlimited water, herb teas, coffee alternatives and
  diluted juice

DAY 3

Breakfast – Fruit yoghurt/yoghurt shake
Lunch – Farmhouse soup
Dinner – Pesto chicken with boiled new potatoes and steamed
  broccoli, raspberry surprise for dessert
Snacks – Two pieces of fruit plus nuts/seeds
Drinks – Unlimited water, herb teas, coffee alternatives and
  diluted juice

DAY 4

Breakfast – Porridge
Lunch – California gold salad with oat cakes

Dinner – Tamale pie with steamed runner beans
Snacks – Two pieces of fruit plus nuts/seeds
Drinks – Unlimited water, herb teas, coffee alternatives and
   diluted juice

DAY 5

Breakfast – Fruit muesli
Lunch – Fatburner baked potato with watercress salad
Dinner – Stuffed aubergines and tomatoes
Snacks – Two pieces of fruit plus nuts/seeds
Drinks – Unlimited water, herb teas, coffee alternatives and
   diluted juice

DAY 6

Breakfast – Fruit yoghurt/yoghurt shake
Lunch – Nutty three bean salad with green salad
Dinner – Kedgeree with steamed courgettes
Snacks – Two pieces of fruit plus nuts/seeds
Drinks – Unlimited water, herb teas, coffee alternatives and
   diluted juice

DAY 7

Breakfast – Scrambled egg with rye toast
Lunch – Stuffed mushrooms
Dinner – Indian spiced chicken with boiled new potatoes and
   steam-fried vegetables, fruit kebabs for dessert
Snacks – Two pieces of fruit plus nuts/seeds
Drinks – Unlimited water, herb teas, coffee alternatives and
   diluted juice

WEEK FOUR

DAY 1

Breakfast – Porridge
Lunch – Fatburner sandwich and rainbow root salad
Dinner – Steamed vegetables and quinoa
Snacks – Two pieces of fruit plus nuts/seeds
Drinks – Unlimited water, herb teas, coffee alternatives and
    diluted juice

DAY 2

Breakfast – Fruit muesli
Lunch – Rice, tuna and bean sprout salad
Dinner – Grilled herring with baked sweet potato and steamed
    spinach
Snacks – Two pieces of fruit plus nuts/seeds
Drinks – Unlimited water, herb teas, coffee alternatives and
    diluted juice

DAY 3

Breakfast – Fruit yoghurt/yoghurt shake
Lunch – Sardines on toast with green salad
Dinner – Tofu steak with buckwheat noodles and steamed
    broccoli, raspberry sorbet for dessert
Snacks – Two pieces of fruit plus nuts/seeds
Drinks – Unlimited water, herb teas, coffee alternatives and
    diluted juice

DAY 4

Breakfast – Porridge
Lunch – Energy soup

Dinner – Roasted chicken breast with brown basmati rice and Mediterranean tomato and broccoli salad (or steamed vegetables)

Snacks – Two pieces of fruit plus nuts/seeds

Drinks – Unlimited water, herb teas, coffee alternatives and diluted juice

DAY **5**

Breakfast – Fruit muesli

Lunch – Fatburner baked potato with watercress salad

Dinner – Grilled burger with rye bread and salad

Snacks – Two pieces of fruit plus nuts/seeds

Drinks – Unlimited water, herb teas, coffee alternatives and diluted juice

DAY **6**

Breakfast – Fruit yoghurt/yoghurt shake

Lunch – Mexican bean dip and crudités

Dinner – Fish pie with steamed courgettes

Snacks – Two pieces of fruit plus nuts/seeds

Drinks – Unlimited water, herb teas, coffee alternatives and diluted juice

DAY **7**

Breakfast – Boiled egg with rye toast

Lunch – Crunchy tofu salad

Dinner – Your choice of steam-fried vegetables with basmati brown rice, peach and carob cream for dessert

Snacks – Two pieces of fruit plus nuts/seeds

Drinks – Unlimited water, herb teas, coffee alternatives and diluted juice

22

Recipes

IF YOU EQUATE healthy food with endless salads and boring bean dishes, the following recipes will prove an extremely pleasant surprise. Each recipe is balanced, according to the principles in this book, to help your metabolism to work properly.

Almost all recipes are sugar-free, using the natural sweetness present in food. They are also high in fibre, so you don't need to add any extra. The foodstuffs used are naturally high in vital vitamins and minerals. I recommend you buy the freshest ingredients, organic if possible, since these tend to contain more nutrients and are chemical-free.

As this diet is mainly based on fresh vegetables, fruits, beans, lentils and wholegrains, with some fish and chicken, you will find it very economical. You may, however, need to vary the fruits and vegetables, depending on what's in season.

Steam-Frying

A few recipes refer to 'steam-frying'. This is quite different from frying or stir-frying, in that the ingredients are essentially steamed rather than fried. The lower temperature of steaming doesn't destroy nutrients as much as frying.

Start with a shallow pan, or a deep frying pan, with a thick base and a lid that seals well. For the purist, oil-free steam-fry, add 2 tablespoons of liquid – either water or vegetable stock, or water down a fraction of the sauce you are going to cook with. Once this is almost boiling, add some vegetables, turn up the heat and put on the lid. The vegetables will sweat and start to cook. After a minute, add the rest of the ingredients. Turn the heat down after a couple more minutes, and steam in this way until cooked.

An alternative steam-fry involves starting off by adding a teaspoon of olive oil to lightly coat the saucepan. Warm the oil, and add the ingredients. As soon as they are sizzling, after a couple of minutes, add 2 tablespoons of water or vegetable stock (or a fraction of the sauce you are going to use) and cook with the lid on. In this way vegetables can be steam-fried using a fraction of the fat used in frying. The shorter time you steam them for, the more taste the vegetables will have.

All lunches and main meals, except for individual portions such as sandwiches, produce quantities for two people. If there's only one of you, halve the sizes or make enough for two meals. Bon appetit!

BREAKFASTS

Breakfast is the most important meal of the day, since your body's sugar level is at its lowest. If you go to work very early, take your breakfast with you and eat it during a break. All recipes are for one person.

GET UP & GO

Get Up & Go is a powdered breakfast drink made by blending skimmed milk or soya milk with a banana and a serving of Get Up & Go. Nutritionally speaking, it is the ultimate breakfast: each serving gives you more fibre than a bowl of porridge, more protein than an egg, more iron than a cooked breakfast and more vitamins and minerals than a whole packet of cornflakes. Every serving gives you at least 100 per cent of every vitamin and mineral and much more of certain key nutrients. For example, you get 1000mg of vitamin C, the equivalent to more than 20 oranges.

Get Up & Go is made from the best quality wholefoods, ground into a powder. The carbohydrate comes principally from apple powder, the protein comes from quinoa, soya and rice flour, the essential fats from ground sesame, sunflower and pumpkin seeds, the fibre from oat bran, rice bran and psyllium husks and the additional flavour from almond meal, cinnamon and natural vanilla.

It contains no sucrose, no additives, no animal products, no yeast, wheat or milk. And it tastes delicious. Each serving, with half a pint of skimmed milk or soya milk and a banana, provides only 283 calories, making it ideal as part of any balanced diet. It is nutritionally superior to any other breakfast choice and is totally suitable for both adults and children. It is fine to have this for breakfast every day, if you choose. If you eat it with a banana, choose a small one that is not too ripe. Low glycemic index alternatives are a soft pear, or a heaped tablespoon of berries. (See Useful Addresses on page 209 for stockists.)

1 serving Get Up & Go
½ pint (300ml) skimmed milk *or* low-fat soya milk
1 banana *or* pear *or* heaped tablespoon of berries

1. Blend milk, fruit and Get Up & Go powder.

FRUIT MUESLI

You can make this delicious muesli yourself, and experiment with different fruit combinations. It tastes best when the oats or rye are soaked overnight in enough water to cover the ingredients.

2oz (55g) oatflakes *or* 1oz (25g) oats and 1oz (25g) ryeflakes
1 serving of fruit – apple, banana, berries, pear
5oz (140g) natural yoghurt
1 dsp ground flax and pumpkin seeds
⅖ pint (220ml) skimmed *or* soya milk

1. Soak the oats/rye overnight.
2. Add skimmed or soya milk.
3. Top with seasonal fruit, yoghurt and seeds.

PORRIDGE

On a cold winter day nothing can be more warming than porridge. Oats contain special factors that are known to promote a healthy heart and arteries, and are full of fibre and complex carbohydrates.

½ pint (300ml) water
½ pint (300ml) skimmed *or* soya milk
2oz (55g) porridge oats
1 tsp honey
1 dsp ground flax and pumpkin seeds

1. Put the water and half the milk in a saucepan and sprinkle in the oats.
2. Bring to the boil and boil for five minutes, stirring all the time.
3. Serve with milk, seeds and a little honey.

FRUIT YOGHURT OR YOGHURT SHAKE

Low-fat, live, natural yoghurt is a first-class food, unlike its commercial counterpart, in which most bacteria have been destroyed in order to allow a longer shelf life. Live yoghurt is packed with good bacteria that have a spring-cleaning effect on your digestive system, as well as being a fine source of protein.

    10oz (250g) very low-fat live yoghurt
    1 tsp honey
    1 serving of fruit – banana, apple, pear, berries, kiwifruit
    1 dsp ground flax and pumpkin seeds

1. Combine all the ingredients. Use any fruit that is in season.
2. If you prefer, make a shake by processing the mix in a blender.

SCRAMBLED EGG

Eggs are rather high in fat but, eaten occasionally as part of a balanced diet, they are a good source of protein and add variety.

    1 large free-range egg
    dash of skimmed *or* soya milk
    1 tbsp fresh parsley, chopped
    small knob of butter

1. Beat eggs with the milk and parsley.
2. Melt the butter in a small saucepan. Pour in the egg mixture. Cook slowly, stirring constantly.
3. Serve with whole rye toast.

BOILED EGG

This simple breakfast makes a wholesome start to the day.

    1 large free-range egg

1. Boil the egg to taste (3–4 minutes for soft boiled).
2. Serve with very lightly buttered wholegrain rye toast.

LUNCHES

These lunches are all quick and easy to prepare. Many can be made and refrigerated. To save time you may want to make enough for two or three days; soups, for example, can be produced in larger batches and frozen. Most of these recipes can easily be taken to work.

FATBURNER SANDWICHES

Fill two slices of rye bread or a wholemeal pitta pocket with any of the following combinations. Eat with a large salad, Coleslaw or Carrot Soup in the Raw (see recipes on pages 185 and 154):

4oz (120g) cottage cheese with a large handful of alfalfa sprouts

6oz (170g) hummus with a large handful of alfalfa sprouts and cucumber slices

1 small, roasted chicken breast (skin removed) and 1 sliced tomato

¾ packet (5½oz/160g) smoked tofu, 1 sliced tomato and a large handful of watercress

2oz (50g) canned salmon *or* tuna in brine, cucumber and a large handful of cress

1 sliced hard-boiled egg with cress, tomato and lettuce

All of these will make a satisfying lunch. Remember to vary what you have – don't go for the same filling everyday. That way you will get a good variety of nutrients. Avoid butter or margarine. If you do need to moisten the bread (which you shouldn't in the case of hummus or cottage cheese), use tahini, which is a delicious sesame seed paste, or a thin layer of hummus.

Fatburner baked potato/sweet potato

Potatoes are often unfairly left out of slimming recipes, but, like a sandwich, a baked potato can be used as a great base for a satisfying lunch. A sweet potato makes a delicious change from the usual varieties. Remember – only have a small potato so that you don't overdo the carbohydrate portion of your meal. Do eat the skins, as they're full of fibre. When making your own, bake them for as short a time as possible, till they are cooked but still firm on the inside. Have them with any of the fillings below and a large salad or Coleslaw (see recipe on page 185).

  2oz (50g) of tuna in brine blended with a teaspoon of cottage cheese
  4oz (120g) low-fat cottage cheese with chives
  6oz (170g) hummus with a handful of alfalfa sprouts
  11oz (300g) baked beans
  1 mug Dahl (see recipe on page 175)
  1 small, roasted chicken breast (no skin), tossed in 1 tbsp yoghurt
    dressing (blended with black pepper and fresh chives or mint)
  5½oz (160g) tofu, tossed in 1 tsp tamari *or* soy sauce

Stuffed mushrooms

Mushrooms are highly nutritious, containing vitamins, minerals and protein.

  20 large button mushrooms
  10oz (250g) smoked tofu
  1 tbsp low-fat natural yoghurt
  4 tbsp fresh parsley, chopped
  2 sticks of celery
  2 spring onions

1. Clean the mushrooms and remove the stalks.
2. Combine the yoghurt, tofu, parsley, mushroom stalks and finely chopped celery and spring onion. Use this mixture to fill the mushroom cups, and serve cold.

TOFU AND AVOCADO DIP WITH CRUDITÉS

This delicious dip allows you to crunch away on a variety of raw vegetables.

> 7oz (200g) soft tofu
> ½ ripe avocado
> 1½oz (40g) cottage cheese
> 1 clove of garlic
> 1 spring onion
> 1 tbsp fresh parsley, chopped
> pinch of paprika
> 1 tsp tamari *or* soy sauce
> black pepper

1. Blend all the ingredients until smooth.
2. Serve with a variety of seasonal crudités – carrots, cucumber, tomato, lettuce, celery, fennel, endive, Chinese leaves, mushrooms, peppers, cauliflower or broccoli (no limit to amount).

RICE, TUNA AND BEAN SPROUT SALAD

Bean sprouts, being vegetables 'in their youth', are incredibly rich in nutrients and high in vitality. You can sprout them yourself, or buy them from a supermarket or healthfood shop.

> 4oz (100g) brown basmati rice, cooked
> 4oz (100g) tuna in brine, drained
> 1 tbsp olive oil
> 1 tsp tamari *or* soy sauce
> juice of half a lemon
> 4oz (100g) bean sprouts
> 1 carrot, chopped
> 1 spring onion, finely sliced

1. Cook rice and allow it to cool.
2. Combine with the other ingredients.

APPLE AND TUNA SALAD

Tuna fish is rich in essential fatty acids as well as other vital nutrients and protein.

> 1 red apple, chopped
> 3oz (80g) tuna in brine, drained
> 2 sticks of celery, sliced
> 1 little gem lettuce, sliced
> 1 large handful bean sprouts
> 1 tbsp low-fat mayonnaise
> 2½oz (70g) natural live yoghurt
> black pepper

1. Drain the tuna fish and combine it with the other salad ingredients.
2. Blend the mayonnaise and yoghurt and mix it into the salad. Season with black pepper.
3. Serve with oat cakes.

NUTTY THREE BEAN SALAD

No foods are better than beans for satisfying your appetite and giving stamina.

> 12oz (350g) mixed beans (haricot, kidney or flageolet), soaked
>   and cooked or canned
> handful of walnuts
> fresh parsley, chopped
> 2 tbsp olive oil
> 2 tsp tamari *or* soy sauce
> juice of 1 lemon
> 4oz (100g) fennel, chopped
> 4 spring onions, finely sliced
> black pepper

1. Combine all the ingredients and serve with a large, mixed salad.

Soup

As a speedy alternative to the suggested soup recipes, you can choose a serving of one of the better quality soups now commercially available, either Baxter's tinned soup or Covent Garden fresh soup. Remember to include a serving of protein if you choose a vegetable soup. And avoid the creamy ones.

Farmhouse soup

Here's a wonderfully warming and easy-to-make meal in itself. You can really make the most of whatever vegetables are in season – going the whole way with a wide variety, or just three or four types. This soup can be liquidised or left as it is. Use potatoes in moderation, as they can thicken the soup too much.

1lb (500g) chopped fresh seasonal vegetables such as potatoes, swede, celeriac, leeks, celery, carrots, broccoli, cabbage
1 medium onion
1 clove of garlic
2 small chicken breasts (cubed) *or* 8oz (240g) pack of Quorn pieces
7oz (225g) tinned tomatoes
1 tbsp olive oil
1 tsp vegetable stock concentrate

1. Steam-fry the onion and garlic in the oil with the chicken or Quorn.
2. Add the vegetables and tomatoes and enough water to cover, plus the vegetable stock paste/powder. Cover and leave to simmer gently on a low heat until the vegetables are cooked, but not mushy.

If you want a much thicker soup to warm up those winter evenings, add a tablespoon of oat flakes at the same time as the water and stir them in well.

CARROT SOUP IN THE RAW

Ever had a hot, raw soup? This soup is made cold and heated gently, keeping all the vitamin and mineral contents intact. It's also full of fibre. Don't overheat it.

    ½lb (225g) carrots
    1½oz (35g) ground almonds
    ¼ pint skimmed *or* soya milk
    1 tsp vegetable stock paste/powder
    ½ tsp mixed herbs, chopped

1. Place the carrots in a food processor and blend them to a purée.
2. Add the other ingredients, and process until mixed.
3. Warm very gently in a pan.

ENERGY SOUP

This soup is blended raw and heated to serve. You can experiment with the same principle to invent other instant, high-energy soups.

    4 medium carrots
    6 broccoli florets
    1 bunch of watercress
    7oz (200g) tofu
    4 tsp Vecon *or* Marigold stock concentrate
    1 dsp tomato purée
    1 tsp spices/herbs to taste
    ¼ pint skimmed *or* soya milk

1. Put all ingredients in a blender and process well.
2. Serve cold or gently heated (do not boil) with oat cakes.

MEXICAN BEAN DIP AND CRUDITÉS

This spicy red bean dip is a great accompaniment to raw vegetables.

6oz (150g) kidney beans, cooked
3oz (85g) cottage cheese
½ tbsp olive oil
¼ onion, finely chopped
1 clove garlic, crushed
1 tbsp yoghurt
pinch of chilli powder

1. Sauté the onion and garlic gently and add the chilli powder. Cool.
2. Blend all the ingredients, adding more yoghurt if necessary, to give a smooth creamy dip.
3. Serve with a mixture of raw vegetable crudités.

HUMMUS

Chick peas, also known as garbanzo beans, have a unique taste which combines well with tahini, a paste of ground sesame seeds. You may prefer to buy ready-made hummus, which is widely available in supermarkets.

7oz (200g) chick peas, cooked or canned
2 cloves garlic, crushed
2 tbsp olive oil
juice of 2 lemons
4 tbsp tahini
cayenne pepper

1. Place all the ingredients in a food processor and blend until smooth and creamy, adding extra water if necessary.
2. Garnish with a little cayenne pepper.

COTTAGE CORN SALAD WITH PUMPKIN SEED DRESSING

The combination of cheese, corn and seeds increases protein quality and tastes delicious.

> 7oz (200g) low-fat cottage cheese
> 1 gem iceberg lettuce, chopped
> ½ small green pepper, sliced
> 1 handful of alfalfa sprouts
> kernels cut from a raw corncob *or* 4oz (100g) frozen corn, cooked very slightly
> 8 cherry tomato halves to garnish

Dressing:

> 1 tbsp ground pumpkin seeds
> 1 tbsp low-fat natural yoghurt
> 1 tsp low-fat mayonnaise
> 1 tsp skimmed milk

1. Combine all salad ingredients.
2. Mix together the dressing ingredients in a bowl.
3. Toss the salad in the dressing.

CALIFORNIA GOLD SALAD

This dish is excellent for unleashing your artistic talent!

> 1 apple
> 1 nectarine, or other seasonal fruit
> 1 kiwifruit
> 8 grapes, deseeded
> juice of half a lemon
> 9oz (240g) cottage cheese
> alfalfa sprouts

1. Slice the fruit and arrange on individual dishes.
2. Sprinkle with lemon juice and top with cottage cheese and alfalfa sprouts.

CRUNCHY TOFU SALAD

This crunchy salad is one of my favourite lunches. It provides not only a colourful variety of vegetables, but also your daily 15g serving of protein. Cauldron Foods' marinated tofu is available in most supermarkets.

11oz (300g) packet marinated tofu (or smoked if preferred)
2 medium carrots, grated
1-inch round of red cabbage, chopped
2 spring onions, finely chopped
2 sticks celery, sliced
4 broccoli florets, chopped
4 tbsp French dressing

1. Combine all the ingredients in a large bowl and season with black pepper.

SARDINES ON TOAST

This may take you back to childhood days. Served with a large salad, sardines on toast make a delicious, healthy meal.

6oz (150g) sardines in brine, drained
4 slices rye bread
2 tomatoes, sliced
2 tbsp olive oil
black pepper

1. Toast bread. Drizzle with olive oil.
2. Place tomato slices and sardines on top and season with black pepper.

MAIN MEALS

Many of the meals below come with a vegetarian option. If the menu suggests a meal you would prefer not to eat, simply choose an alternative. Some recipes can be prepared in advance and frozen.

STEAM-FRIED VEGETABLES WITH . . .

This dish can be prepared with a variety of ingredients and different seasonings. Choose one of the protein-rich foods, and one of the seasonings, to combine with vegetables.

Vegetables:
Choose from spring onions, garlic, carrots, broccoli, courgettes, cauliflower, sugar snap peas, runner beans, water chestnuts, mushrooms, bean sprouts, peppers, bamboo shoots – enough to fill half your plate.

Protein-rich foods:
11oz (300g) tofu, cubed
or 4oz (100g) chicken, cubed
or 11oz (300g) tempeh, cubed
or 5oz (140g) filleted fish, cubed

Seasoning:
Thai: fresh chopped coriander, green curry paste and a dash of
    coconut milk plus onion and garlic
Chinese: tamari *or* soy sauce, ginger, onion and garlic
Mexican: onion, garlic and watered down Mexican spice sauce
    (from a jar)
Mediterranean: onion, garlic and ½ tin tomatoes with mixed herbs
Indian: onion, garlic and tomatoes with fresh chopped coriander,
    cumin and chilli powder

1. Steam-fry onion and garlic in the chosen seasoning.
2. Add the protein-rich food and steam-fry until cooked.
3. Add a little water and the vegetables. Simmer until the vegetables are cooked but still crunchy.

FISH PIE

This is my favourite fish recipe. Be sure to ask for colouring-free smoked haddock. Smoked haddock should never be bright yellow (the dyes used are no good for you).

100g combined white fish and colouring-free smoked haddock
¼oz (5g) butter
½ tbsp wholemeal flour
2½fl oz (75ml) skimmed *or* soya milk
2½oz (75g) prawns
2oz (50g) button mushrooms
½ tsp mixed herbs
black pepper
¾lb (350g) potato, mashed with a little milk
1 tbsp sesame seeds

1. Steam the fish for 15 minutes.
2. Make a white sauce using the butter, flour and milk.
3. Combine the fish, sauce, prawns, mushrooms and herbs. Place in an ovenproof dish and top with the mashed potatoes. Sprinkle with sesame seeds.
4. Bake for 30 minutes at 200°C/400°F/gas mark 6.

You can experiment with different types of fish or seafood – maybe a variety including cod, haddock, salmon or even mussels, scallops or squid. For a slightly unusual hint of flavour, you may like to grate a little nutmeg into the white sauce.

KEDGEREE

It is important not to overcook brown rice. Apart from the fact that it will be stodgy and unpleasant, it will be transformed from a complex into a simple carbohydrate. The rice should still be in separate grains and not have the appearance of splitting out of its skin. Use twice the quantity of boiling water to rice, and simmer, covered, until all the water is absorbed.

    5oz (140g) colouring-free smoked haddock
    4oz (100g) brown basmati rice
    ½ pint (325ml) water
    1 free-range egg
    fresh parsley, chopped
    paprika

1. Bring the water to the boil in a saucepan. Add the rice and boil for 25 minutes with the lid tightly on.
2. Meanwhile steam the haddock in a little water.
3. Combine the flaked haddock and rice.
4. Hard boil the egg. Slice, and add it to the haddock and rice. Garnish with parsley and paprika.

CHICK PEA CRUMBLE

Chick peas are an excellent food. They can be bought dry, soaked overnight and cooked. Alternatively, tinned chick peas are already cooked.

Filling:
1 small onion, chopped
1 tsp olive oil and 2 tbsp water
¼ red pepper, chopped
1 stick of celery
2 medium carrots, chopped
7oz (200g) tinned tomatoes
14oz (400g) canned chick peas
pinch of cumin

Crumble:
4oz (100g) wholemeal flour
2oz (50g) butter
1oz (25g) oats
1 tbsp pumpkin seeds

1. Steam-fry the onion, celery, red pepper and carrots.
2. Add the other ingredients and simmer for 20 minutes.
3. Rub butter into the flour. Mix in the oats and pumpkin seeds.
4. Place the filling in an ovenproof dish and top with the crumble.
5. Bake at 190°C/375°F/gas mark 5 for 30 minutes.

If you're not really a great fan of chick peas, you could use another bean such as borlotti, navy, butter beans or even a mixture. Many supermarkets now sell such mixes in cans. If you do use canned beans, be sure to rinse and drain them well as they are often in salted water.

SHEPHERDESS PIE

This vegetarian equivalent of shepherd's pie is easy to make and very tasty. Soya mince, which is available dried in most supermarkets, is a very convincing alternative to minced meat – most meat-eaters don't notice any difference. If you prefer, you can use turkey mince instead.

1 tsp olive oil and 2 tbsp water
1 small onion, chopped
1 clove of garlic, crushed
7oz (200g) canned tomatoes
75g dried soya mince *or* 4oz (100g) turkey mince
1 tbsp parsley, chopped
1 tbsp tamari *or* soy sauce
¾lb (350g) mashed potato
1 tbsp sesame seeds

1. Steam-fry the onion and garlic in the oil.
2. Add the tomatoes, parsley, aduki beans and tamari. Simmer gently for 15 minutes.
3. Place the bean mixture in an ovenproof dish and top it with mashed potatoes and sesame seeds.
4. Bake for 35 minutes at 200°C/400°F/gas mark 6.

SWEET AND SOUR STEAM-FRY

This Chinese-style dish has a delicious Oriental taste. The combination of the sauce ingredients makes for a wonderfully contrasting taste – on the one hand enticing your sweet taste buds, yet on the other, giving them a sharp tang.

1 tsp olive oil and 2 tbsp water
1 clove of garlic, chopped
½ onion, chopped
½ green pepper, chopped
1 carrot, sliced
½ tin of pineapple chunks (unsweetened, in own juice)
11oz (300g) tofu *or* 4oz (100g) skinless chicken breast, cubed

Sauce:
2 tsp cornflour
4 tbsp pineapple juice
3 tbsp cider vinegar
1 tbsp brown sugar
2 tsp tamari *or* soy sauce
1 tbsp tomato purée

1. Steam-fry the chicken in the oil for 5 minutes, until cooked through.
2. Add the vegetables. (If using tofu recipe, start by steam-frying the vegetables in oil.)
3. Combine the sauce ingredients and add them to the vegetables, together with the pineapple and tofu, if used. Simmer for 3 minutes, stirring well.

The carrot, pepper and onion is perfect for this dish, but if you like, you can experiment with a different selection of vegetables such as broccoli, mangetout and baby sweetcorn.

TAMALE PIE

This Mexican-style recipe is made of a bean and chilli pot topped with cornbread.

1 tsp olive oil and 2 tbsp water
1 small onion, chopped
1 clove of garlic, chopped
pinch of chilli powder
¼ green pepper, chopped
4oz (100g) kidney beans
4oz (100g) turkey mince *or* 3oz (75g) dried soya mince (soaked) *or*
    9oz (240g) Quorn mince
7oz (200g) tinned tomatoes

Topping:
2oz (65g) cornmeal
½ tbsp wholemeal flour
1 tsp baking powder
1 free-range egg, beaten
1¾fl oz (50ml) skimmed milk

1. Steam-fry the onion, garlic and pepper with the chilli powder.
2. Add the mince, kidney beans and tomatoes and simmer for 5 minutes.
3. Blend the cornmeal, flour and baking powder. Beat in the egg, milk and oil to produce a thick batter.
4. Place the bean and chilli mix in an ovenproof dish. Spoon the cornbread mixture over it.
5. Bake at 220°C/425°F/gas mark 7 for about 40 minutes until golden.

GRILLED BURGERS*

Many supermarkets now stock good ready-made vegetarian burgers and sausages. Choose the ones without hydrogenated fat or additives. But here is a healthy, home-made, vegetarian alternative to the hamburger.

8oz (220g) tofu, mashed
4 tbsp tamari *or* soy sauce
1 medium carrot, grated
1 clove of garlic, crushed
1 small spring onion, chopped
2 slices of rye bread, toasted and crumbed
1 tbsp tomato purée
1 medium-sized free-range egg
black pepper
1 tbsp fresh coriander, chopped
1 tbsp olive oil

1. Mix the tofu and soy sauce in a bowl. Leave for 20 minutes, then squeeze out and discard any excess moisture.
2. Mix all the ingredients except the oil in a bowl. Form the mixture into 4 burgers. Chill for 20 minutes.
3. Lightly brush the burgers with oil. Grill under a medium grill for 15 minutes, turning frequently.
4. Serve between two slices of rye bread, with sliced tomato and lettuce.

*Courtesy of Cauldron Foods.

There's nothing like picking up a burger with your hands and tucking into it (if you can get your mouth round it!). It may even take you back to the bad old days when you slipped into the fast food burger joints. No need for that now you've got a great-tasting, healthy alternative.

CHICKEN SALAD

Chicken contains half the fat of other meats.

cold meat cut from half a small roast chicken, without the skin
1 large eating apple, cubed
2 sticks of celery, chopped
5oz (140g) cold boiled potatoes, cubed
1 tbsp low-fat mayonnaise
1 tbsp low-fat yoghurt
1 tsp horseradish sauce
2 tbsp skimmed milk
1 gem lettuce
red pepper to garnish

1. Create a bed of lettuce on a large plate.
2. Combine all ingredients except the pepper, and pile them on top of the lettuce.
3. Decorate with rings of red pepper on top.

MUSHROOM PILAF

Mushrooms can be eaten raw in salads, or cooked, as in this delicious pilaf. The secret is to cook them slowly. Adding a little water helps to bring out their juices.

2oz (60g) brown basmati rice
1 tbsp olive oil
1 small onion, chopped
¼ pint hot water
¼ red pepper, diced
11oz (300g) smoked tofu, cubed
1½oz (50g) frozen peas
2oz (60g) mushrooms, sliced
½ tsp Vecon *or* Marigold stock concentrate
½ tsp finely chopped root ginger
1 tbsp fresh parsley, chopped

1. Gently heat the oil in a heavy frying pan. Fry the rice in it until pale brown. Add the onion and cook for a further 5 minutes.
2. Add the water, pepper and mushrooms. Cover and simmer until the liquid is absorbed and the rice is just tender. Add more hot water if needed.
3. Stir in the stock, tofu and ginger.
4. Cook the frozen peas. Drain and add to rice mixture.
5. Serve garnished with the parsley.

SPICY MACKEREL WITH COUSCOUS

The North African hint in this spicy sauce complements mackerel well, and calls for couscous, an excellent source of carbohydrate that is very easy to prepare.

    2 small mackerel fillets
    1 tsp olive oil and 2 tbsp water
    1 small onion, finely chopped
    1 clove of garlic, crushed
    1 red pepper, chopped
    4oz (110g) courgettes, sliced
    ¼ tsp chilli powder
    1 tsp cumin powder
    7oz (200g) tinned tomatoes
    4oz (115g) couscous
    ¾ pint (440ml) boiling water

1. Place the mackerel fillets in a baking tray, cover and bake for 20 minutes.
2. Pour the boiling water over the couscous. Leave it to stand for 15 minutes.
3. Meanwhile, steam-fry the onion, garlic, cumin and chilli powder for 2 minutes.
4. Add the courgettes and red pepper and sauté for a further 2 minutes.
5. Add the tomatoes and simmer until the vegetables are tender but still crisp.
6. Arrange a fish fillet on a mound of couscous. Top with the sauce.

CHILLI

This wonderful dish has often fooled a hardy meat-eater. It is another dish which can be prepared in double quantity and frozen.

1½oz (50g) dried soya mince *or* 6½oz (180g) Quorn mince
1 tsp olive oil and 2 tbsp water
½ green pepper, sliced
1 small onion, sliced
2 cloves of garlic, crushed
½ tsp chilli powder
1 tsp paprika
1 tsp ground cumin
1 tsp ground coriander
7oz (200g) canned tomatoes, chopped
1 tbsp tomato purée
4oz (110g) canned kidney beans

1. Steam-fry the onions, garlic and pepper in the oil with the chilli, cumin and coriander.
2. Add the pre-soaked mince or Quorn and stir for 2 minutes.
3. Add the tomatoes, tomato purée and kidney beans. Mix well and leave to simmer for at least half an hour, stirring occasionally to prevent the bottom from burning. If the mixture becomes too thick, add a little water.

A big pot of this chilli can go a long way – it's tasty, satisfying and warming. It's even something you could serve all your friends, providing all the usual condiments that go with it such as guacamole (avocado dip), salsa (spicy tomato dip), sliced lettuce and sour cream.

SPAGHETTI MARINARA

Use whatever seafood you fancy in this dish. A variety works best. Some supermarkets sell a frozen mix, or you could make your own selection. You can easily double the quantity of the sauce and freeze half of it for another time.

If you've never tried wholewheat or buckwheat spaghetti, this is the recipe to try either with. I prefer buckwheat spaghetti, but you have to be a bit careful how you cook it. Bring it to the boil, then add cold water and bring it back to the boil. Do this twice for best results.

6oz (150g) wholewheat *or* buckwheat spaghetti
1 small onion, chopped
2 cloves of garlic, crushed
1 tsp olive oil and 2 tbsp water
½ green pepper, chopped
1 tbsp tomato purée
7oz (200g) canned tomatoes
6oz (150g) mixed seafood (fresh prawns, mussels, fish, squid, tinned clams)
1 tsp concentrated vegetable stock
½ tsp fresh thyme, chopped

1. Steam-fry the onion and garlic in the oil.
2. Add the green pepper and seafood and sauté for 5 minutes.
3. Add the vegetable stock, thyme, tomato purée and tinned tomatoes. Cover and leave to simmer for 20 minutes. Add a little water if the sauce gets too thick.
4. Cook the spaghetti in plenty of boiling water for about 12 minutes, then drain.
5. Serve the spaghetti topped with the sauce.

Spaghetti bolognese

This is a vegetarian variety of the classic Italian dish. It can be prepared in batches and frozen, for convenience.

> 3oz (75g) dry soya mince *or* 9oz (240g) Quorn mince
> 1 small onion, chopped
> 2 cloves of garlic, crushed
> 1 tsp olive oil and 2 tbsp water
> 14oz (400g) canned tomatoes
> 1 tbsp tomato purée
> 2 bay leaves
> ½ tsp mixed herbs
> 1 tsp Vecon *or* Marigold stock concentrate
> 2 tbsp red wine

1. If using soya mince, presoak it (follow the instructions on the packet).
2. Steam-fry the onions and garlic in the oil and herbs for 2 minutes. Add the mince and tomato purée and stir for a further 3 minutes.
3. Add the tomatoes, stock concentrate, red wine and bay leaves. Stir well.
4. Cover and leave to simmer for at least half an hour. Stir occasionally to make sure the bottom is not burning. If it starts to thicken too much, add a little water. If you find it's too watery, leave the lid off.
5. Serve with wholewheat spaghetti or other pasta shapes.

Pasta Provençale

Provençale dishes conjure up a sense of my childhood days spent in southern France. This one is a quick favourite.

11oz (300g) smoked tofu *or* 2 small chicken breasts, diced
1 small onion, chopped roughly
1 tsp olive oil and 2 tbsp water
2 cloves of garlic, crushed
1 green pepper, chopped
1 small courgette, chopped
1 aubergine, cubed
7oz (200g) canned tomatoes
1 tsp tomato purée
1 tsp Vecon *or* Marigold stock concentrate
1 tsp mixed fresh herbs

1. Steam-fry the onions and garlic for 2 minutes before adding the chicken or tofu. Then add the chopped vegetables, tomatoes, tomato purée, vegetable stock concentrate and herbs.
2. Cover and leave to simmer for 20 minutes.
3. Serve over freshly cooked wholewheat pasta shapes.

The particularly 'Provençale' flavour comes from that great Mediterranean mix of vegetables – garlic, peppers, aubergines, courgettes and tomatoes as well as the fresh herbs. If you can't get hold of fresh herbs, use a dried blend.

THAI BAKED COD

Thai seasoning is subtle and delicious. You can use any white fish instead of cod if you prefer, and the dish tastes even better if the fish is left to marinate in the sauce for a few hours before cooking. It goes very well with the Crunchy Thai Salad (see page 184).

> 2 2½oz (70g) cod fillets
> juice and grated zest of 1 lime
> ½ inch ginger root, grated
> 1 stick of lemon grass, sliced
> 2 cloves of garlic, crushed
> 1 tsp tamari *or* soy sauce
> 1 fresh chilli, finely chopped

1. In a mug, blend the lime juice, lime zest, lemon grass, crushed garlic, tamari and chilli. Beware – when you chop chilli, wash your hands immediately, as the oil from it can burn if you rub your eyes or other sensitive parts of your body.
2. Rinse the cod fillets and place them in a baking dish.
3. Pour the lime mixture over the fish, turning it so it is well coated.
4. Cover with a lid or foil and bake in a preheated oven (200°C/400°F/gas mark 6) for 20 minutes (or until cooked – this will depend on the thickness of the fish).

ROAST CHICKEN

Organic, free-range chicken is the best. Once you've roasted the chicken, remove the skin before eating. Leftover meat can be used to make sandwiches the next day.

 1 medium chicken
 ½ lemon
 1 dsp tamari

1. Rub the tamari and the juice of the lemon all over the chicken. Place the squeezed-out lemon half inside the chicken cavity.
2. Put the chicken in a roasting dish and bake in a preheated oven (190°C/375°F/gas mark 5), calculating 20 minutes per pound.

POACHED SALMON

With its unique flavour, salmon is often best cooked simply, with little seasoning.

 2 2oz (55g) salmon fillets
 2 lemon wedges
 black pepper

1. Place the rinsed salmon in a steamer and steam for 15–20 minutes, depending on the thickness of the fillets. Alternatively poach the fish by placing it in a baking dish with a tablespoon of water. Cover it and bake for 20 minutes.
2. Serve with lemon wedges and black pepper.

INDIAN SPICED CHICKEN

For this dish, it's fun to experiment with different combinations of spices. You could even just use a ready-made curry powder.

> 2 2oz (50g) chicken breasts
> juice of 1 lemon
> ½ tsp turmeric powder
> ½ tsp ground cumin
> 1 tsp ground coriander
> dash of cayenne
> 1 clove of garlic, crushed

1. Blend the lemon juice, garlic and spices.
2. Place the rinsed chicken in a dish and toss it in the spice blend until it is well coated. Leave to marinate for at least 30 minutes, or ideally several hours.
3. Place under a hot grill for 25 minutes, or until cooked. This will depend on the thickness of the chicken. Turn it once, halfway through cooking.

GRILLED PESTO CHICKEN

This dish has a wonderful Mediterranean taste and is well complemented by the Mediterranean Tomato and Broccoli Salad (see page 184).

> 2 2oz (50g) skinless chicken breasts
> 1 heaped tsp ready-made pesto

1. Slice the rinsed chicken breasts across and spread their insides with half of the pesto.
2. Spread the remaining pesto on top of the chicken.
3. Grill for 25 minutes, or until cooked. This will depend on the thickness of the chicken.

DAHL (LENTIL CURRY)

This dish – a favourite of mine – is a variation on a recipe given to me by a woman from Goa. Despite the lentils, it always goes down well with meat-eaters. Leftovers can be frozen or eaten with a baked potato for lunch the following day.

11oz (300g) orange lentils
3½ mugs of water
1 medium onion, chopped
4 cloves of garlic, chopped
14oz (400g) canned tomatoes
1 heaped tsp curry powder
1 tsp Vecon *or* Marigold stock concentrate

1. Rinse the lentils well in cold, running water until the water runs clear.
2. Place in a saucepan with the water, onions and garlic.
3. Bring to the boil and simmer for 20 minutes.
4. Add the curry powder, stock concentrate and tomatoes and stir well. Cover and leave to simmer for a further 30 minutes, stirring occasionally to make sure the bottom does not burn. If it starts to get too thick, add a little water. If it seems too watery, leave uncovered.

THAI GREEN CURRY

This dish has a wonderfully aromatic blend of spices and can be made with any one of the protein-rich foods listed below. Green curry paste, fish sauce and kaffir lime leaves are now widely available in some supermarkets and Asian grocery shops. If you can't find the last two, the curry should still taste great without them.

2 2oz (50g) chicken breasts, cubed *or* 11oz (300g) firm tofu, cubed *or* 6oz (170g) peeled prawns
1 small onion, chopped
2 cloves of garlic, crushed
1 tsp olive oil and 2 tbsp water
2 heaped tsp green curry paste
1 dsp fish sauce
1 large courgette, chopped
2 kaffir lime leaves
handful of fresh basil leaves
400ml canned coconut milk

1. Steam-fry the onions, garlic and curry paste in oil for 2 minutes.
2. Add the chicken/tofu/prawns and fry for a further 5 minutes.
3. Add the coconut milk and kaffir lime leaves. Stir well, cover and leave to simmer for at least half an hour.
4. Add the courgettes and basil leaves 5–10 minutes before serving.

You may like to experiment with a variety of vegetables – green beans are widely used in Thailand as are mushrooms, which add to the great contrast in textures.

STUFFED AUBERGINES AND TOMATOES

These provide a delicious, full meal in themselves. Green or red peppers and marrows can be used as alternatives.

1 large aubergine
2 large tomatoes
1 tsp olive oil and 2 tbsp water
1 small onion, finely chopped
1 clove garlic, crushed
11oz (300g) smoked tofu, finely chopped *or* 4oz (100g) turkey
     mince *or* 9oz (240g) Quorn mince
1 tsp Vecon *or* Marigold stock concentrate
2oz brown basmati rice, cooked
handful of fresh parsley, chopped
1 heaped tsp mixed herbs
black pepper
1 tsp olive oil, to grease tray

1. Cut the aubergine in half lengthways and scoop out the inside flesh. Cut the tops off the tomatoes and scoop out the seeded flesh. Place the aubergines on the greased tray and bake in a preheated oven (190°C/375°F/gas mark 5) for 20 minutes. Meanwhile, steam-fry the onion and garlic in the oil for 2 minutes. Add the turkey or tofu, fry for a further 5 minutes before adding the scooped-out vegetable flesh and stock concentrate. Add 2–3 tablespoons water and leave to simmer for 3 minutes.
2. In a large bowl, combine the cooked tofu/turkey/Quorn and vegetables with the rice and parsley. Season with black pepper.
3. Remove aubergines from oven (leave it on). Stuff them, and the tomatoes, with the mixture.
4. Place them back on the baking tray. Bake in the oven for 35 minutes.

ROAST VEGETABLES WITH QUINOA AND HARISSA

With its high-protein content, quinoa is a remarkable food. In this dish, it is complemented well by the roasted vegetables. The spicy sauce is a variation on the North African harissa.

8oz (225g) quinoa
1½ pints (860ml) water
10 cherry tomatoes
1 medium carrot, sliced
1 medium courgette, cubed
1 red pepper, sliced
4 button mushrooms
1 medium onion, cut into 8
2 dsp olive oil

Harissa:
2 peeled plum tomatoes, fresh or canned
¼ tsp cayenne pepper
1 tsp cumin powder
1 tsp coriander powder
1 clove of garlic
dash of vinegar

1. Place all the vegetables on a baking tray and lightly drizzle with olive oil.
2. Bake in a preheated oven (180°C/350°F/gas mark 4) for 50 minutes. Remove twice during cooking to shake tray to turn and recoat vegetables.
3. Meanwhile, rinse the quinoa thoroughly under cold, running water. Place it in a saucepan with the water. Bring to the boil, cover and simmer for 13 minutes, or until the water is absorbed.
4. Place the harissa ingredients in a blender to form a paste. Add vinegar if the paste is too stiff.
5. Serve a mound of quinoa topped with vegetables and a little harissa on the side.

STEAMED VEGETABLES WITH QUINOA

The idea of steamed vegetables may sound bland, but the dressing in this recipe turns them into a delicious, light feast.

1 medium onion, sliced into rounds
1 clove of garlic, sliced
4 broccoli florets, chopped
1 medium carrot, chopped
10 runner beans, sliced
8oz (225g) quinoa
1½ pints (860ml) water

Dressing:
2 dsp sesame oil
1 tsp tamari
squeeze of lemon juice
black pepper

1. Rinse the quinoa thoroughly under cold, running water. Place it in a saucepan with the water. Bring to the boil, cover and simmer for 13 minutes or until the water is absorbed.
2. Mix the dressing ingredients in a cup.
3. Place the onion, garlic and carrots in a vegetable steamer and steam for 5 minutes. Add the broccoli and beans and steam for a further 5 minutes. Take care not to overcook the vegetables. (This will depend on the size of the pieces.)
4. Serve the vegetables on a mound of quinoa. Pour over the dressing.

The dressing here makes a world of difference. If you are not keen on sesame oil, use extra virgin olive oil or another cold pressed seed oil instead.

TOFU STEAK

This is a delicious way to eat tofu, together with vegetables or perhaps some brown basmati rice, or buckwheat noodles.

11oz (300g) of either smoked tofu or marinated tofu pieces
finely sliced vegetables choosing from carrots, beansprouts, sugar
    snap peas, mangetout, broccoli pieces or green pepper

Sauce:
4 tbsp soup stock *or* vegetable stock
1 tbsp tamari *or* soy sauce
1 tsp of pear and apple spread
1 tsp grated ginger
6 finely sliced shiitake mushrooms
1 tbsp apple juice

1. Combine the sauce ingredients and simmer in a saucepan until thickening but still runny. If necessary add 1 tsp of corn starch.
2. Add either the smoked tofu or the marinated tofu and the vegetables to the sauce and simmer for 2 minutes, stirring so that the tofu absorbs the sauce.
3. Serve on brown basmati rice or buckwheat noodles.

This recipe will get rid of any preconceptions that a pile of tofu sounds rather unappealing. In this recipe the sauce conjures up a strong taste of the East and the shiitake mushrooms give your immune system a good boost.

ROAST CHICKEN BREAST

This is a delicious, easy dinner to prepare.

    2 small chicken breasts (with skin)
    1 dsp olive oil
    1 clove of garlic, sliced
    two sprigs of fresh tarragon
    ½ lemon

1. Place the garlic slices and tarragon under the chicken skin.
2. Place chicken breasts in a baking dish and drizzle with olive oil and lemon juice.
3. Place in an oven preheated to 190°C/375°F/gas mark 5. Bake for 20 minutes or until cooked (this will depend on the thickness of the chicken). Before eating, remove the skin.

GRILLED HERRING

Herrings are one of the best fish for providing omega-3 essential fats as well as protein and vitamins. The flavour is strong and needs little enhancement.

    1 5oz (150g) herring
    half a lemon
    black pepper

1. Squeeze the juice of the lemon and grind the black pepper over the herring. Place it under a medium grill for 20 minutes. Turn halfway through cooking.

SALADS AND DRESSINGS

Several of the salads given in the lunch suggestions have a dressing to go with them.

FRENCH DRESSING

This standard French dressing can be jazzed up with fresh and dried herbs. Also experiment with other oils such as cold-pressed sesame oil or flax oil, which contain essential fatty acids. Use as little dressing as possible on salads.

> 3 tbsp olive oil
> 1 tbsp Essential Balance or Udo's Choice (see Useful Addresses on
>   page 209)
> 2 tbsp cider vinegar *or* balsamic vinegar
> 1 tsp French mustard
> 1 clove garlic, crushed

1. Put all the ingredients in a screw-top jar and shake vigorously. Any leftover dressing can be stored in the fridge.

TAHINI DRESSING

The crushed sesame seeds and oil in tahini make a dressing thicker and creamier.

> *either*
> 2 tbsp home-made French dressing
> 1 tbsp tahini
> *or*
> 1 tsp honey
> 1 tsp mustard
> 2 tbsp Essential Balance *or* Udo's Choice
> 1 tbsp tahini
> juice of ½ lemon

1. Put all the ingredients in a screw-top jar and shake vigorously. Any extra dressing can be stored in the fridge.

WATERCRESS SALAD

Watercress is rich in iron and vitamin A. It is delicious in salad.

½ bunch watercress
1 gem lettuce, sliced
¼ cucumber, sliced
½ green pepper, chopped
1 handful of alfalfa sprouts

1. Combine all the ingredients and toss with 1 tbsp French or tahini dressing.

GREEN SALAD

This simple green salad is a good accompaniment to any meal.

⅓ Cos or other lettuce, chopped
¼ bulb of fennel, sliced
4 broccoli florets, chopped
¼ cucumber, chopped
2 sticks of celery, sliced

1. Combine all the ingredients and toss them with 1 tbsp French dressing.

MEDITERRANEAN TOMATO AND BROCCOLI SALAD

Conjure up a taste of Italy with this great combination of soft tomatoes and crunchy broccoli. If you can find them, use real Italian plum tomatoes instead of cherry tomatoes.

10–15 cherry tomatoes, halved
6 medium broccoli florets, chopped
6 large, fresh basil leaves, roughly torn
1 dsp olive oil
2 tsp balsamic vinegar
black pepper

1. Toss all the ingredients together.

CRUNCHY THAI SALAD

This is a variation on one of the most popular street food dishes in Thailand, where it is made to order – in a mortar and pestle – and never in advance. It originally comes from the northeast of the country, but it is now available in your own kitchen!

¼ medium white cabbage, finely shredded
8 runner beans, sliced
1 medium tomato, chopped
1 chilli, very finely chopped
juice of 2 limes
1 dsp fish sauce
1 dsp apple juice
1 handful of peanuts, roughly crushed

1. Combine all the ingredients in a large bowl and toss well. If you are not keen on hot food, leave out the chilli, or be careful not to eat the pieces once they have flavoured the salad.

TOMATO AND SPROUTED BEAN SALAD

Sprouted beans – such as mung beans, aduki beans, lentils and chick peas – are highly nutritious and can either be bought or sprouted at home.

1 beef tomato, diced
5oz (140g) sprouted beans
3 finely chopped spring onions
1 dsp extra virgin olive oil
juice of ½ lemon
black pepper
small handful of chopped fresh basil

1. Toss all the ingredients together.

COLESLAW

Cabbages are packed with vitamins and minerals, and so are carrots, high in vitamin A, and onions, high in sulphur containing amino acids, which help to remove toxins from the body.

7oz (200g) red or white cabbage, finely shredded
3oz (200g) carrots, grated
½ small onion, finely chopped
1 tbsp low-fat mayonnaise
1 tbsp very low-fat live yoghurt
½ tbsp skimmed milk

1. Mix all the ingredients well in a large bowl.

RAINBOW ROOT SALAD

This colourful combination of carrots, parsnips and beetroots is more filling than you would imagine. Go easy on the beetroot and parsnips – their strong taste can overpower the carrots.

2 medium carrots, grated
1 small parsnip, grated
1 small beetroot, grated
handful of parsley, finely chopped
1 tbsp olive oil
1 tbsp lemon juice
black pepper

1. Combine all the ingredients and toss well.

DESSERTS

APRICOT WHISK

This dessert tastes even better than it looks. Using dried apricots, rich in micronutrients, it can be made all year round.

4oz (110g) apricots
¼ tsp natural vanilla essence
5oz (140g) low-fat natural yoghurt
3oz (80g) cottage cheese
1 egg white

1. Stew apricots until soft. (Soak overnight, if using dried apricots.)
2. Blend in a processor, adding the vanilla essence, yoghurt and cottage cheese.
3. Whisk the egg white stiffly. Fold into the apricot mixture.
4. Place in a bowl or individual glasses. Chill before serving.

FRESH FRUIT SALAD

The addition of one or two interesting fruits improves a fruit salad enormously. Try mango, kiwifruit, fresh lychee, strawberries, fresh dates or melon.

1lb (450g) mixed fruits
1oz (25g) dried apricots
4 tbsp natural yoghurt

1. Cut the fruit into cubes.
2. Stew apricots and liquidise, adding enough water to make a pourable sauce.
3. Pour the cooled sauce and natural yoghurt over the fruit.

RASPBERRY SURPRISE

This fruit fool is also delicious made with strawberries or black-currants.

8oz (225g) raspberries (fresh, or frozen and thawed)
4oz (100g) low-fat fromage frais
1–2 tsp honey
handful of fresh mint leaves

1. Blend raspberries, fromage frais and honey.
2. Pour into individual serving dishes. Garnish with a sprig of mint.

DRIED APRICOTS WITH CASHEW CREAM

This wonderful dessert always goes down a treat. It is quite rich, so watch out!

4oz (110g) dried apricots
1oz (25g) whole hazelnuts
3oz (80g) cashew nuts

1. Soak the apricots in boiling water. When soft, remove their stones and replace them with whole hazelnuts.
2. Grind the cashews in a blender until fine. Slowly trickle in water to produce a cream-like consistency.
3. Serve the apricots with the cashew cream, arranged in a sundae glass.

Rhubarb and Blackcurrant Pie

If you like rhubarb, you'll love the combination of rhubarb and blackcurrant in this pie.

8oz (220g) rhubarb
4oz (110g) blackcurrants
¼ tsp ground ginger
4oz (110g) cottage cheese
⅛ pint (75ml) skimmed milk
½ tbsp honey
2 tbsp ground almonds

1. Stew the rhubarb and blackcurrants in a small amount of water until soft. Mix in the ginger and put in ovenproof dish.
2. Mix the cottage cheese, milk and honey together thoroughly. Cover the fruit with the cheese mixture.
3. Sprinkle with almonds. Toast lightly under a hot grill.

You can use any fruit that takes your fancy, or whatever is in season. One traditional combination – apple and blackberry – goes very well with the topping. In this case, some cinnamon and a few cloves added makes a delicious alternative. In the summer you could try a mixture of seasonal berries.

FRUIT KEBABS

This is a light, refreshing dessert that goes down well after any main meal. You can experiment with other fruits – just check what's in season.

> 1 green apple
> 1 red apple
> 1 banana
> juice of 1 lemon
> 1 orange
> 6 black grapes
> 7oz (200g) natural yoghurt
> 1 tsp honey

1. Cube the apples and banana. Coat with a little lemon juice to prevent them from going brown. Peel the oranges, removing all the pith, and cut into chunks. Halve the grapes and remove the pips.
2. Put the fruit onto skewers, and grill under a high grill or on a barbecue.
3. Blend the yoghurt with honey and use as a dipping sauce.

RASPBERRY SORBET

There are many variations to this theme, which allow you to pick fruit in season, and freeze and use it whenever you want. Just think – raspberries and strawberries all year round!

> ½lb (225g) frozen raspberries
> 1 banana, chopped into ½-inch lengths
> 4 tbsp natural yoghurt
> sprigs of mint

1. Freeze the bananas.

2. Remove the bananas and raspberries from the freezer and allow them to partially thaw (about 5 minutes).

3. Blend fruit with yoghurt in a food processor. Serve immediately in sundae glasses, decorated with a sprig of mint.

PEACH AND CAROB CREAMS*

You can serve these to impress guests if you are entertaining. Otherwise they make a delicious, sweet treat anyway.

4oz (110g) tofu
7oz (200g) can peaches in juice
3 tsp honey
½ medium banana
¼ pint cold water
1 tsp agar agar (available from healthfood stores)
2 tsp carob powder (available from healthfood stores)
small carob bar, grated

1. Liquidise the tofu, peaches and juice, honey and banana.

2. Blend the water, agar agar and carob powder in a small saucepan. Bring it to the boil, stirring constantly. Pour the mixture into the liquidiser and blend it until smooth.

3. Transfer to one large, or four individual, dishes and chill.

4. Decorate with the grated carob bar.

*Courtesy of Cauldron Foods

DRINKS AND SNACKS

The following drinks can be consumed without limit throughout the day:

water
herb teas
dandelion coffee, Barleycup, Caro, Teechino

The following drinks are best limited to three glasses a day:

Aqua Libra and other sugar-free juice blends (best diluted)
fruit juices, diluted 50 per cent with water

Limit alcohol to a maximum of 5 units a week, although 3 is better and none is best. The following are each 1 unit:

a small glass of wine
a half-pint of beer or lager
a measure of spirits

The only snacks allowed are two pieces of fruit each day choosing from: apples, pears, plums, cherries, berries, peaches, grapefruit, oranges, grapes and tangerines.

It is fine to eat a banana with a low GI cereal such as oats or Get Up & Go, but not as an additional snack. It is best to take your two fruit snacks mid-morning and mid-afternoon, away from your main meals. If you haven't had your full quota of essential fats from other sources also take the equivalent of 1 dessertspoon of pumpkin seeds with each fruit snack.

APPENDIX 1

Your Ideal Weight and Body Fat Percentage

The Ideal Weight for Your Height

The following tables show your ideal weight range depending on your height and sex.

Men aged 25 and over		Women aged 25 and over	
Height	Weight (lb)	Height	Weight (lb)
5′1″	112–129	4′8″	92–107
5′2″	115–133	4′9″	94–110
5′3″	118–136	4′10″	96–113
5′4″	121–139	4′11″	99–116
5′5″	124–143	5′0″	102–119
5′6″	128–147	5′1″	105–122
5′7″	132–152	5′2″	108–126
5′8″	136–156	5′3″	111–130
5′9″	140–160	5′4″	114–135
5′10″	144–165	5′5″	118–139
5′11″	148–170	5′6″	122–143
6′0″	152–175	5′7″	126–147
6′1″	156–180	5′8″	130–151
6′2″	160–185	5′9″	134–155
6′3″	164–190	5′10″	138–159

Body Fat Percentage

A more important statistic than your 'ideal weight' is your Body Fat Percentage. The following equation allows you to work out an approximation of your Body Fat Percentage. (Your local gym may offer the service of measuring your Body Fat Percentage more accurately using callipers or testing equipment.) An ideal Body Fat Percentage for a man is less than 15 per cent and for a woman, less than 22 per cent. You can reduce your Body Fat Percentage by around 10 per cent a month on the Fatburner Diet.

Step 1

Find your Body Weight (BW) on the chart on page 195 and write down the corresponding Conversion Factor. For weights which are not multiples of 5lb, take the figure below your weight and add 1.08 to the Conversion Factor for every pound over it. For example:

If you weigh 175lb, your Conversion Factor is 189.36

If you weigh 132lb, your Conversion Factor is 142.83 $(140.67 + [2 \times 1.08])$

Step 2

Find your Waist Girth on the chart and write down the corresponding Conversion Factor. For example:

If you have a 35-inch waist, your Conversion Factor is 145.26

Step 3

Subtract the Waist Conversion Factor from the Body Weight Conversion Factor. For example:

$189.36 - 145.26 = 44.10$

Step 4

Men add 98.42 to the result. Women add 76.76. This gives your Lean Body Weight (LBW). For example:

$44.10 + 98.42 = 142.52$

Step 5
To calculate your Fat Weight (FW), subtract the LBW from the BW. For example:

175 − 142.52 = 32.48

Step 6
To determine your Body Fat percentage, divide FW by BW and multiply by 100. For example:

(FW/BW) × 100 = %BF.

(32.48/175) × 100 = 19%

Body fat percentage calculation chart

Body weight	Conversion factor	Waist girth	Conversion factor
100	108.21	25	103.75
105	113.62	25.5	105.83
110	119.03	26	107.9
115	124.44	26.5	109.98
120	129.85	27	112.05
125	135.26	27.5	114.13
130	140.67	28	116.2
135	146.08	28.5	118.28
140	151.49	29	120.35
145	156.9	29.5	122.43
150	162.31	30	124.51
155	167.72	30.5	126.58
160	173.13	31	128.66
165	178.54	31.5	130.73
170	183.95	32	132.81
175	189.36	32.5	134.88
180	194.77	33	136.96
185	200.18	33.5	139.03

chart continues

Body weight	Conversion factor	Waist girth	Conversion factor
190	205.59	34	141.11
195	211	34.5	143.18
200	216.41	35	145.26
205	221.82	35.5	147.33
210	227.23	36	149.41
215	232.64	36.5	151.48
220	238.05	37	153.56
225	243.46	37.5	155.63
230	248.87	38	157.71
235	254.28	38.5	159.78
240	259.69	39	161.86
245	265.1	39.5	163.93
250	270.51	40	166.01
255	275.92	40.5	167.08
260	281.33	41	170.16
265	286.74	41.5	172.23
270	292.15	42	174.31
275	297.56	42.5	176.38
280	302.97	43	178.46
285	308.38	43.5	180.53
290	313.79	44	182.61

APPENDIX 2

Monitoring Your Progress and Fatburner Research

Follow the instructions in Chapter 20 to monitor your progress week by week using the Fatburner Progress Report on the following pages. There's a Progress Report for each of the first four weeks, and a spare Progress Report to be copied for subsequent weeks.

FATBURNER PROGRESS REPORT

WEEK No. 1   Starting date: / /   Ending date: / /

THIS WEEK

Initial weight _____ Bust/chest _____ Waist _____ Hips _____ Thighs _____

Final weight _____ Bust/chest _____ Waist _____ Hips _____ Thighs _____
(at end of week)

Target weight _____ Bust/chest _____ Waist _____ Hips _____ Thighs _____

PROGRESS THIS WEEK

Weight lost _____ Total inch loss _____

How many aerobic sessions? _____ How many toning sessions? _____

How well did you follow the diet? _____ % the exercises? _____ %

PROGRESS TO DATE

Initial weight _____ Initial total inches _____
(at start of diet)   (bust+waist+hips+thighs)

Weight lost to date _____ Inches lost to date _____

FATBURNER PROGRESS REPORT

WEEK No. 2   Starting date: / /   Ending date: / /

THIS WEEK

Initial weight _____ Bust/chest _____ Waist _____ Hips _____ Thighs _____

Final weight _____ Bust/chest _____ Waist _____ Hips _____ Thighs _____
(at end of week)

Target weight _____ Bust/chest _____ Waist _____ Hips _____ Thighs _____

PROGRESS THIS WEEK

Weight lost _____ Total inch loss _____

How many aerobic sessions? _____ How many toning sessions? _____

How well did you follow the diet? _____ % the exercises? _____ %

PROGRESS TO DATE

Initial weight _____ Initial total inches _____
(at start of diet)   (bust+waist+hips+thighs)

Weight lost to date _____ Inches lost to date _____

FATBURNER PROGRESS REPORT

WEEK No. 3   Starting date: /   /   Ending date: /   /

THIS WEEK

Initial weight _____ Bust/chest _____ Waist _____ Hips _____ Thighs _____

Final weight _____ Bust/chest _____ Waist _____ Hips _____ Thighs _____
(at end of week)

Target weight _____ Bust/chest _____ Waist _____ Hips _____ Thighs _____

PROGRESS THIS WEEK

Weight lost _____ Total inch loss _____

How many aerobic sessions? _____ How many toning sessions? _____

How well did you follow the diet? _____ % the exercises? _____ %

PROGRESS TO DATE

Initial weight _____ Initial total inches _____
(at start of diet) (bust+waist+hips+thighs)

Weight lost to date _____ Inches lost to date _____

FATBURNER PROGRESS REPORT

WEEK No. 4   Starting date: /   /   Ending date: /   /

THIS WEEK

Initial weight _____ Bust/chest _____ Waist _____ Hips _____ Thighs _____

Final weight _____ Bust/chest _____ Waist _____ Hips _____ Thighs _____
(at end of week)

Target weight _____ Bust/chest _____ Waist _____ Hips _____ Thighs _____

PROGRESS THIS WEEK

Weight lost _____ Total inch loss _____

How many aerobic sessions? _____ How many toning sessions? _____

How well did you follow the diet? _____ % the exercises? _____ %

PROGRESS TO DATE

Initial weight _____ Initial total inches _____
(at start of diet)   (bust+waist+hips+thighs)

Weight lost to date _____ Inches lost to date _____

FATBURNER PROGRESS REPORT

WEEK No. ☐   Starting date: / /   Ending date: / /

THIS WEEK

Initial weight _____ Bust/chest _____ Waist _____ Hips _____ Thighs _____

Final weight _____ Bust/chest _____ Waist _____ Hips _____ Thighs _____
(at end of week)

Target weight _____ Bust/chest _____ Waist _____ Hips _____ Thighs _____

PROGRESS THIS WEEK

Weight lost _____ Total inch loss _____

How many aerobic sessions? _____ How many toning sessions? _____

How well did you follow the diet? _____ % the exercises? _____ %

PROGRESS TO DATE

Initial weight _____ Initial total inches _____
(at start of diet)   (bust+waist+hips+thighs)

Weight lost to date _____ Inches lost to date _____

FATBURNER RESEARCH QUESTIONNAIRE

You can help with ongoing Fatburner research. If you've completed the diet for four or more weeks, let us know your results by filling in this simple questionnaire, answering as many questions as you can and sending or faxing it to: Fatburner Research, 34 Wadham Road, London SW15 2LR (fax: 0181 874 5003).

Your full name _____

Address _____

_____

Contact number _____

What was your initial weight? _____ lb/kg

How many weeks did you/have you follow(ed) the Fatburner Diet? _____

What was your final weight? _____ lb/kg

Bust/chest _____ Waist/Hips _____ Thighs _____ inches/cm

Body fat percentage _____ (if known)

How well did you follow the diet indications? _____ %

How well did you follow the exercise indications? _____ %

How easy was the diet to follow? easy ☐ reasonable ☐ hard ☐
very hard ☐

How did you find the recipes? excellent ☐ good ☐ fair ☐
not good ☐

Did you mainly follow the rules or the recipes? _____ % (half and half would be 50/50)

How did you feel while on the diet? _____

_____

_____

Did you notice any other changes to your health? _____

_____

What do you think made the biggest difference? _____

_____

Any other comments? _____

_____

Working Out Your Training Heart Rate Zone

The best way to know that you are exercising at an intensity that will burn fat and boost your metabolism is to measure your pulse while exercising. If it is within your Training Heart Rate Zone for 15 minutes or more then you are having a fatburning effect.

To find your training heart rate zone, you need to subtract your age from 220, then calculate 65% of this amount for the lower end of your training zone and 80% for the upper limit:

$$220 - \text{Age} \_\_ \times .65 = \text{lower limit}$$
$$220 - \text{Age} \_\_ \times .80 = \text{upper limit}$$

For example, for a 30 year old:

$$220 - 30 = 190 \times .65 = \text{lower limit} = 124 \text{ beats per min}$$
$$220 - 30 = 190 \times .80 = \text{upper limit} = 152 \text{ beats per min}$$

To find your pulse rate, you will need a watch with a second hand. There are several points at which the pulse can be felt easily: the neck (the Carotid pulse) on either side of the Adam's apple; or the wrist (the radial pulse). To find your pulse, apply light pressure with your fingers. Normally, for medical examinations your pulse is taken for 60 seconds. But to find your pulse while exercising, stopping for this long would lower your pulse and give you a false reading. So taking your pulse for only 10 seconds and multiply the result by 6 will give you the number of beats in one minute without giving your heart rate a chance to slow down. This will be your exercising pulse rate.

When you first embark on your aerobic exercise sessions, you will need to stop briefly every 10–15 minutes to monitor your pulse. After a while you will become familiar with how the correct pulse feels for you. See the chart below to find your exercise heart rate for your age.

Training Heart Rate Zone Chart (while exercising)

Age (beats in 1 minute)	65–80% of maximum heart rate (beats in 10 sec.)	
20	130–160	22–27
22	129–158	22–26
24	127–157	21–26
26	126–155	21–26
28	125–154	21–26
30	124–152	21–25
32	122–150	20–25
34	121–149	20–25
36	120–147	20–25
38	118–146	20–24
40	117–144	20–24
45	114–140	19–23
50	111–136	19–23
55	107–132	18–22
60	104–128	17–21
65	101–124	17–21
70	98–120	16–20

The centre column shows how many beats you should have in one minute. Beginners should aim for the lower figure on the left hand side (that is, 65% of their maximum heart rate for their age). Then slowly increase to 80% of their maximum heart rate. Do not exceed this higher level. The column on the far right gives you how many beats you should have in a 10 second pulse count. Beginners should stay at the lower end of their exercise range.

References

Part 1

1. MAFF National Food Survey (1977–97).
2. ORIC Press Release January 1998.
3. ORIC; McArdle, W. *Medical Aspects of Clinical Nutrition*, Keats 1983.
4. Appelbaum, N. *Influences of level of energy intake on energy expenditure in man.*
5. Leibel, R. et al. 'Changes in energy expenditure resulting from altered body weight.' *NEngl J Med*, 1995; 332: 621–628.
6. Wynn, M. & A. 'How dieting can damage your health.' *Which? Way to Health*, February 1995, pp. 22–24.
7. Allen, L. et al. 'Protein-induced hypercalcuria: a longer term study.' *Am J Clin Nutrition*, 1979; 32: 741–749; Anand, C. et al. 'Effect of protein intake on calcium balance of young men given 500mg calcium daily.' *J of Nutrition*, 1974; 104: 695–700.
8. Gittlemann, Ann Louise *Beyond Pritikin*, New York, Bantam, revised edition 1996.
9. Hull, H. 'The Effect of Food Combining on Weight Loss.' ION research project, 1997.
10. Wynn, op cit.
11. Maconaghie, P. 'A comparison of the metabolic diet with the Unislim diet for inducing weight loss.' ION (1988).

Part 2

12. Reaven, G. 'Role of Insulin Resistance in Human Disease.' *Diabetes*, 1988; 37: 1595–1607.
13. Wolever, T. *The Glycemic Index.*

14. Rankins, J. 'Glycemic Index and Exercise Metabolism.' *Gatorade Sports Science Institute Sport Science Exchange*, 1997; 10(1).

15. Heaton, K. et al. 'Particle size of wheat, maize and oat test meals: effects on plasma glucose and insulin responses and on the rate of starch digestion in vitro.' *Am J Clin Nutrition*, 1988; 47: 675–82.

16. Wolever, T. et al. 'Beneficial effect of low-glycemic index diet in overweight NIDDM subject.' *Diabetes Care*, 1992; 15(4): 562–564; Jenkins, D. et al. 'Low-glycemic index diet in hyperlipidemia: use of traditional starchy foods.' *Am J Clin Nutrition*, 1987; 46: 66–71.

17. Reaven, op cit.

18. Jenkins, D. et al. 'Glycemic index of foods: a physiological basis for carbohydrate exchange.' *Am J Clin Nutrition*, 1981; 34: 362–366.

19. Garg, A. 'High monounsaturated fat diets for patients with diabetes mellitus: a meta-analysis.' *Am J Clin Nutrition*, 1998; 67(suppl): 577S–582S.

20. Bolton-Smith, C. et al. 'Dietary composition and fat to sugar ratios in relation to obesity.' *Int J Obesity*, 1994; 18: 820–8.

21. Delargy, H. et al. 'Effects of amount and type of dietary fibre (soluble and insoluble) on short-term control of appetite.' *Int J Food Sciences and Nutrition*, 1997; 48: 67–77.

22. Kissilef, H. *Am J Phys*, 1980; 238: 14–22; Konnyyaku *S Agr Biol Chem*, 1970; 34(4): 641–643; Matsuura, M. *Jap Diabetic Assoc*, 1980; 23(3): 209–217.

23. Mito, A. Data held in ION library, source unknown.

24. Walsh, D. Unpublished study at GNC Research Center, Fargo, North Dakota (1982).

25. Holford, P. 'The Effects of Glucomannan on Weight Loss.' ION (1983).

26. *The Vitamin Controversy Report*, ION (1987).

27. Wunderlich, R. *Sugar and Your Health*, Good Health Publications, Florida (1982).

28. Davies, S. 'Zinc, Nutrition & Health' *Yearbook of Nutritional Medicine* (1984/5).

29. Davies, S. et al. 'Age-related decreases in chromium levels in 51,665 hair, sweat and serum samples from 40,872 patients – implications for the prevention of cardiovascular disease and type II diabetes mellitus.' *Metabolism*, 1997; 46(5): 1–4.

30. Evans, G. 'The effect of chromium picolinate on insulin controlled parameters in humans.' *Int J Biosocial & Med Research*, 1989; 1(2): 163–180.

31. Riales, R. et al. 'Effects of chromium chloride supplementation on

glucose tolerance and serum lipids including high density lipoprotein of adult men.' *Am J Clin Nutrition*, 1981; 34: 2670–2678; Abraham, A. et al. 'The effects of chromium supplementation on serum glucose and lipids in patients with and without non-insulin-dependent diabetes.' *Metabolism*, 1992; 41: 768; Glinsmann, W. et al. 'Effects of trivalent chromium on glucose tolerance.' *Metabolism*, 1966; 15: 510–515; Levine, R. et al. 'Effects of oral chromium supplementation on the glucose tolerance of elderly human subjects.' *Metabolism*, 1968; 17: 114–124; Hambidge, K. 'Chromium: A Review.' *Disorders of Mineral Metabolism, vol 1: Trace Minerals* pp. 272–94, Academic Press (1981).
32. Mervyn, L. *Report on Minerals*, (unpublished), JWT client report.
33. Colgan, M. *Your Personal Vitamin Profile*, Blond & Briggs (1983).
34. Clouatre, D. and Rosenbaum, M. *The Diet and Health Benefits of HCA*, Keats Publishing (1994).
35. Prentice, A. and Jebb, S. 'Obesity in Britain: gluttony or sloth?' *BMJ*, 1995; 311: 437–9.
36. McArdle, W. *Medical Aspects of Clinical Nutrition*, Keats (1983).
37. Broughton, D. et al. 'Review Deterioration of Glucose Tolerance with age: The Role of Insulin Resistance.' *Age and Ageing*, 1991; 20: 221–225.
38. Wald, D. *Health & Fitness* magazine.
39. Hollenbeck, C. et al. 'Effect of habitual exercise on regulation of insulin stimulated glucose disposal in older males.' *J Am Geriatr Soc*, 1986; 33: 273–7.

Further supporting research is available from the Lambert's Library at the Institute for Optimum Nutrition (ION), see page 209), whose members are free to visit and study there. ION also offers information services, including literature and library search facilities, for readers who would like to access scientific literature on specific subjects. On page 211, you will find a list of the best books to use to follow up information given in *The 30-Day Fatburner Diet*.

Useful Addresses

Essential Oil Blends containing a combination of cold-pressed seed oils are becoming more widely available. The best two products are Essential Balance, distributed by Higher Nature (see below) and Udo's Choice, distributed by Savant Distribution, 7 Wayland Croft, Adel, Leeds, West Yorkshire LS16 8LA (tel: 0113 2301993).

Health Plus produces an extensive range of supplements – including konjac fibre (glucomannan) – available by mail order. Send for a free catalogue to Health Plus Ltd., Dolphin House, 30 Lushington Road, Eastbourne, East Sussex BN21 4LL (tel: 01323 737374).

Higher Nature produces a wide range of supplements including HCA and chromium. They also supply Get Up & Go. Send for a free colour catalogue and newsletter to Higher Nature, Burwash Common, East Sussex TN19 7LX (tel: 01435 882880).

The Institute for Optimum Nutrition offers personal consultations with qualified nutrition consultants and runs courses including the one-day Optimum Nutrition Workshop, the Homestudy Course and the three-year Nutrition Consultants' Diploma Course. It also has a Directory of Nutrition Consultants (£2) which will help you find a nutrition consultant in your area. For a free information pack, write to: ION, Blades Court, Deodar Road, London

SW15 2NU (tel: 0181 877 9993; fax: 0181 877 9980; website: **www.optimumnutrition.co.uk**).

Nutrition Consultation. For a personal referral by Patrick Holford to a clinical nutritionist in your area specialising in weight management, please write to Holford & Associates, 34 Wadham Road, London SW15 2LR. Enclose your name, address, telephone number and brief details of your health issue. Alternatively visit his website: **www.patrickholford.com**

Psychocalisthenics is an excellent exercise system that you can do at home in under 20 minutes. Either learn in a day at trainings held throughout the UK, or follow a teaching video and book. For further details contact MetaFitness, Squires Hill House, Tilford, Surrey GU10 2AD (tel: 01252 782661).

Solgar produces an extensive range of supplements, including HCA and chromium, available through healthfood shops. For your nearest stockist, contact Solgar Vitamins Ltd., Aldbury, Tring, Hertfordshire HP23 5PT (tel: 01442 890355).

Recommended Reading

Chapter 4
Kathleen Des Maisons, *Potatoes not Prozac*, Simon & Schuster (1998)
Anthony Leeds, Jennie Brand Miller, Kaye Foster-Powell and Stephen Colagiuri, *The GI Factor*, Hodder & Stoughton (1996)
Leighton Steward, Morrison Bethea, Sam Andrews and Luis Balart, *Sugar Busters*, Ballantine Books (1995)

Chapter 5
Patrick Holford, *Beat Stress and Fatigue*, Piatkus (1999)
Patrick Holford, *100% Health*, Piatkus (1998)

Chapter 6
Barry Sears Ph.D., *Enter The Zone*, Regan Books (1995)

Chapter 7
Udo Erasmus, *Fats that Heal, Fats that Kill*, Alive Books (1987, revised 1994)

Chapter 9
Patrick Holford, *The Optimum Nutrition Bible*, Piatkus (1997)

Chapter 10
Stephen Langer and James Scheer, *Solved: The Riddle of Illness*, Keats (1984, revised 1995)
Kate Neil and Patrick Holford, *Balancing Hormones Naturally*, Piatkus (1998)

Chapter 12
Gloria Thomas, *Apples & Pears*, Orion (1998)

Index

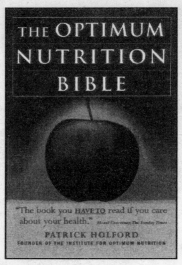

0 7499 1748 2 (HB)/0 7499 1855 1 (PB)   352pp   £14.99 (HB)/£10.99 (PB)

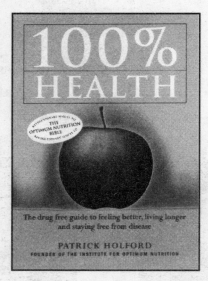

0 7499 1813 6 (HB)   224pp   £14.99 (HB)

All Optimum Nutrition titles available from good bookshops. Alternatively contact Piatkus Books, Customer Services Department on 0171 631 0710 or on the 24-hour freephone number, 0800 454816.

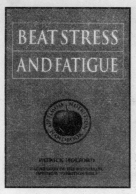

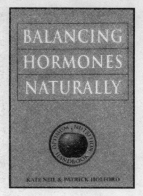

0 7499 1952 3 (PB)   160pp   £5.99

0 7499 1863 2 (PB)   192pp   £5.99

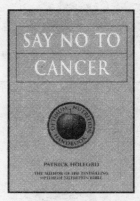

0 7499 1953 1 (PB)   160pp   £5.99

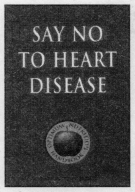

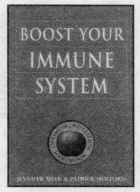

0 7499 1862 4 (PB)   160pp   £5.99

0 7499 1864 0 (PB)   192pp   £5.99